Etiological Explanations

Etiological Explanations
Illness Causation Theory

Olaf Dammann
Professor and Vice Chair
Public Health and Community Medicine
Tufts University School of Medicine
Boston, Massachusetts, USA
and
Professor
Department of Gynecology and Obstetrics
Hannover Medical School
Hannover, Germany

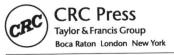

CRC Press
Taylor & Francis Group
Boca Raton London New York

CRC Press is an imprint of the
Taylor & Francis Group, an **informa** business

First edition published 2020
by CRC Press
6000 Broken Sound Parkway NW, Suite 300, Boca Raton, FL 33487-2742

by CRC Press
2 Park Square, Milton Park, Abingdon, Oxon, OX14 4RN

© 2020 Taylor & Francis Group, LLC
CRC Press is an imprint of Taylor & Francis Group, LLC

Library of Congress Cataloging-in-Publication Data

Names: Dammann, Olaf, author.
Title: Etiological explanations : illness causation theory / by Olaf Dammann.
Description: First edition. | Boca Raton : CRC Press, [2020] | Includes bibliographical references and index.
Identifiers: LCCN 2019056063 | ISBN 9781498784290 (paperback) | ISBN 9780367471309 (hardback) | ISBN 9780429184147 (ebook)
Subjects: MESH: Pathologic Processes--etiology | Epidemiologic Methods
Classification: LCC RC69 | NLM QZ 140 | DDC 616/.047--dc23
LC record available at https://lccn.loc.gov/2019056063

ISBN: 978-1-4987-8429-0 (pbk)
ISBN: 978-0-367-47130-9 (hbk)
ISBN: 978-0-429-18414-7 (ebk)

Visit the Taylor & Francis Web site at
http://www.taylorandfrancis.com

and the CRC Press Web site at
http://www.crcpress.com

For Christiane

CONTENTS

PREFACE

Epidemiology, the science of the determinants of illness in populations, lacks a comprehensive theoretical framework for the metaphysics and epistemology of causation. In this book, support is offered for the argument that it is possible, and perhaps even useful, to move from causal inference to *etiological explanation in epidemiology*. In particular, a proposal is made that etiological pluralism is pluralism of causes and of causation, and that it requires the consideration of different kinds of causal and mechanistic evidence. Further, it is argued that a process perspective will be helpful when looking at the combined contribution of etiological factors. Finally, it is argued that explanatory coherentism might be a viable framework for comprehensive etiological explanations.

This book has been many years in the making. The first versions of the idea date back to 1994 when I visited the Chapel Hill campus of the University of North Carolina. My wife and pediatrician colleague Christiane participated in a workshop there, which gave me two days in the campus library. It was there that I developed the nested bicone model of illness causation (see Section 2.4.2 in this book). The manuscript I wrote about it was never published, so the idea sees the light of day only now, more than 25 years later.

I have read philosophical texts, in particular philosophy of science, since my high school days. Many years later, with formal degrees in medicine and epidemiology, I still read anything I can lay my hands on in the area of causation and causal inference. In 2014, I discovered to my great excitement Alex Broadbent's book *Philosophy of Epidemiology* and submitted a book review about it to the journal *Philosophy of Science*. I contacted Alex, he graciously listened to my amateurish questions, and he helped me *a lot* to grasp the nuances of his book. I found out that his academic home, the University of Johannesburg in South Africa, offers a master's degree track in philosophy that builds on a research project, and I asked Alex if he would accept me as a student with a project about etiological explanations. I was thrilled when he agreed and suggested to wrap my thesis around a series of published articles. Two years and 80,000 words into the project, we decided to transition from a master's to a doctoral thesis, which I submitted in October 2018. This book is an updated, considerably modified, and expanded version of that thesis. Thanks once more for all your help and guidance, Alex.

I work in an academic field that does not encourage the publication of books but almost exclusively values publications of articles in scholarly journals. Perhaps as a consequence of this fact, and of my difficulty producing longer, coherent texts, I began writing articles about the theory of etiology in epidemiology. One of the earliest was coauthored with Alan Leviton; I will always be grateful for his mentorship and collegial guidance, and for his unlimited enthusiasm for the good cause of preventing brain damage among the most vulnerable newborns. Some of the more recent articles form the backbone of individual chapters in this book. I would like to thank Carmina Erdei and Alex Fiorentino for allowing me to recycle some of the material we coauthored, and James Marcum, Martha Montello, Alfredo Morabia, and Gregory Radick for chaperoning some of these pieces toward publication. Special thanks to my editor at CRC Press/Taylor & Francis Group, Jo Koster, for guidance and patience. I am grateful to all others who offered helpful direct or indirect input for those papers, my thesis, and this book: Alex Broadbent, Ryan Flanagan, Jeremy Howick, Ted Poston, Federica Russo, David Spurrett, Paul Thagard, Jan Vandenbroucke, Jon Williamson, and multiple anonymous reviewers. My apologies to those I am omitting here inadvertently.

Most importantly, I thank my wife Christiane and our daughters Lina and Laura. Neither this book nor I would be without them.

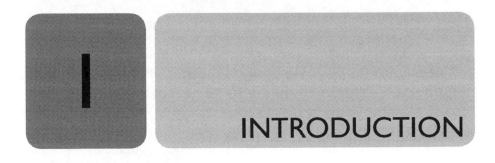

INTRODUCTION

Sitting appears to be the new smoking. According to the CNN Health News website,

> a growing amount of research suggests that just standing – even if you don't walk around – can have health benefits.[1]

The research that triggers such news is brought to you by epidemiologists. In this field of health research, scientists collect information on a large number of individuals from well-defined populations. Then, they attempt to identify patterns of risk factors for health outcomes, based on the observation of processes that begin with the *exposure* to a putative cause of illness (e.g., smoking) and end with the *outcome*, the occurrence of disease (e.g., lung disease). Their stated goal is to identify causes of illness. By doing so, they contribute to a narrative that details the story of illness occurrence. They help generate *etiological explanations*.

1.1 WHAT THIS BOOK IS AND IS NOT ABOUT

A close look at what epidemiologists do day in, day out suggests that their primary goal is to identify modifiable risk factors with the intention to intervene in ways that help prevent, or at least reduce, the occurrence of adverse health events in populations (Tulchinsky and Varavikova 2009:41–3). This goal has led to the notion that in order to be able to talk about an observed *statistical association* between risk factors (exposures) and health outcomes as a *causal association*, some kind of tool is needed to help with causal inference based on observed data.

Current epidemiology employs two very different tools to do just that. The first is a quantitative tool called the *potential outcomes approach* (POA). It postulates that (a) "in ideal randomized experiments, association is causation" (Hernan and Robins 2006a:578) because (b) "the randomized experiment [is] the only scientifically proven method of testing causal relations from data" (Pearl 2000:340). The POA is based on three main assumptions. First, it is rooted in counterfactual reasoning (as in "had the exposure not occurred, the outcome had not occurred"). Second, it holds that randomization is the closest we can get to a scenario that allows us to formally test counterfactual *causal* hypotheses. Obviously, a direct observation of counterfactuals is impossible because we cannot directly observe, for example, what would have happened if the patient who took the drug and got better had not taken it.[2] Third, the POA holds that in situations where randomization is impossible, quasi-randomization can emulate it, and results from such observational studies can be interpreted as indicative of a causal relationship (Imbens and Rubin 2015).

The POA is not discussed in this book, but instead the focus is on the second, qualitative tool available to epidemiologists. In 1965, Sir Austin Bradford Hill published the speech he gave on January 14 of that year before the Section of Occupational Medicine of the Royal Society of Medicine in the United Kingdom. In this paper, Hill listed nine points that he thought would be helpful to ponder when looking at the results of an observational (nonrandomized) study (Hill 1965). Among these are, for example, the strength of the association, whether or not there is a dose-response relationship between exposure and outcome, and how well the observed result fits with the rest of the available knowledge. Taken together, these nine viewpoints can be thought of as a scaffolding for comprehensive explanations of why certain illnesses occur. This is what I call an *etiological explanation,* the concept at the core of this book. Part of my discussion explicates my observation that the way Hill's heuristics are used in epidemiology is well-aligned with the philosophical concepts of *explanatory coherentism* (Poston 2014) and *evidential error independence* (Claveau 2012).

Thus, my overarching goal is to offer an account of *etiology of illness* and of *etiological explanation.* The question I want to tackle is, "What is etiology and what do health scientists get out of it?" This book offers a descriptive account of the schism between epidemiological and basic science accounts of how illness comes about. It is also an account of how the *textbook goal* of epidemiology, that is, identifying causes of illness by describing exposure-outcome relationships, can morph into its *de facto goal,* that is, providing *useful etiological explanations.*

At first approach, *etiology* is depicted as "the cause, set of causes, or manner of causation of a disease or condition" (Google) or even simpler, "the cause of a disease or abnormal condition" (Merriam-Webster). Epidemiologists state, in accordance with these commonsensical definitions, that they intend to find *causes.* What they are actually doing, however, looks more like an effort to find more holistic explanations of disease occurrence that go beyond the identification of mere causes. Such explanations go beyond listing the causes in a disease's natural history. It is the attempt to tell etiological stories that include the why (causes) *and* the how (pathogenesis) of illness, bringing the presence or absence of causes together with their functional consequences, their pathogenetic effects. When adequately satisfying something like these conditions, a story about how a case of illness comes about is an *etiological explanation* of that case. I hold that while the POA restricts one to making causal inferences based on observational data, etiological explanations offer far more.

Epidemiologists can more or less ignore the contents of the black box between exposure and outcome, because successful prevention does not rely on pathogenetic knowledge. All it takes is knowledge about risk factors that are candidate causes, the modification of which is likely to result in changes in illness occurrence. In contrast, basic science explanations zoom in on that black box, which contains the pathogenetic process that connects exposure and outcome, the biological process that is initiated by the exposure and results in disease occurrence. Both are ways to explain illness occurrence, that is, causal and pathogenetic explanations.[3] I suggest unifying causal and pathogenetic explanations under the heading *etiological explanations*. The reason why etiological explanations work for us is because they are holistic descriptions of the natural history of illness, provided in a single narrative that integrates new data with background knowledge, either by linking causes to pathogenetic processes, or vice versa, depending on the time frame and sequence of discovery. This suggestion resonates with Salmon's account of etiological explanation and with Lewis' theory of causal explanation as providing information about causal histories. It also resonates with unificationist accounts of scientific explanation (Friedman 1974; Kitcher 1981, 1989). However, neither of these accounts features prominently in views of causation already implemented in epidemiology, which mainly derive from Mill (reflected in Hill) and Mackie (reflected in Rothman).[4]

1.2 ROAD MAP

This book is based on a series of papers published between 2014 and 2018 for which I was either a sole author (Dammann 2015, 2016, 2017, 2018) or the coauthor of one of my trainees (Erdei and Dammann 2014). Each chapter following the second is based on one of these papers. Although each chapter stands on its own and can be read without much background needed from reading the previous ones, they all speak to particular aspects of the overarching question of how etiological explanations are constructed. One of these papers is published in a philosophy journal (*Philosophy of Science*), one in an epidemiological journal (*American Journal of Epidemiology*), and three in interdisciplinary journals (*Theoretical Medicine and Bioethics* and *Perspectives in Biology and Medicine*). This variety of journals underlines the notion that this is an *interdisciplinary* book in the philosophy of epidemiology. My task is not an entirely philosophical one but one that requires me to reach across the divide between philosophy and the sciences. It is not first philosophy, but it employs an interdisciplinary approach that allows me to draw on both the epidemiological and philosophical literature and to offer arguments based on techniques of reasoning from both fields. This represents a continuous challenge, a constant risk that I am running from the perspective of readers who come from only one of the disciplines involved. Similarly, the mark of success for this book is not defined by one discipline alone. Instead, the hope is that both philosophers and epidemiologists will consider this book a valuable contribution to their interdisciplinary discourse.

Chapter 2: A Multidisciplinary Problem. The next chapter introduces some crucial concepts and approaches. First offered is a brief introduction to epidemiology, the science that helps explain the occurrence of illness. Next, the concept of etiology is introduced as the telling of the story of illness occurrence, and some terminology is clarified. The topics of epidemiological metaphysics and epistemology round off this chapter.

Chapter 3: Etiological Explanations. This is an essay review (Dammann 2015) of Alex Broadbent's book *Philosophy of Epidemiology* (Broadbent 2013). In it, I first review the text from the epidemiological perspective and accept Broadbent's invitation to move from causation and causal inference to explanation. I offer thoughts on a possible extension of Broadbent's proposal for what is a good causal inference. In essence, inference and confirmation by intervention are conceptualized as one possible way to make etiological explanations even better by making them more useful. In the postscript, I contrast epidemiologists' textbook goals (what they say they do, i.e., find causes of illness) and their de facto goals (what they are actually doing quite well, i.e., contribute to useful etiological explanations). That suggestion is then expanded to consider *explanation by intervention* as one way to improve etiological explanations.

Chapter 4: Etiological Pluralism. This chapter is based on an essay review (Dammann 2016) of Phyllis Illari and Federica Russo's text on causality in the health sciences, in which they provide an overview of causal inference techniques (Illari and Russo 2014). I discuss their claim that a mosaic of such techniques should allow for good causal explanations and suggest that this does not seem particularly useful unless we agree on a schema of *how* to integrate evidence gathered in multiple ways from multiple sources. I also propose that etiological pluralism is pluralism about the real-world phenomenon of the illness causation process, not about various concepts of it.

Chapter 5: Difference-Making and Mechanism. The theme of *useful* etiological explanations from Chapter 3 is picked up here. Federica Russo and Jon Williamson have suggested that causal claims in the health sciences need support from both difference-making and mechanistic evidence. This proposal has come to be known as the Russo–Williamson thesis (RWT). I summarize and discuss the arguments from four papers by Russo and Williamson that support the RWT and offer a review of previous critiques, including my own.

Chapter 6: Process Perspective. Causation and causal inference are of utmost importance in my field of expertise, developmental neuroepidemiology. One prominent example is autism causation. A unified model of autism causation remains elusive. Therefore, well-designed explanatory models are needed to develop appropriate therapeutic and preventive interventions. In the paper that forms the basis of this chapter, Carmina Erdei and I have argued that autism is not a static disorder but rather an ongoing process (Erdei and Dammann 2014). I discuss the link between preterm birth and autism and briefly review the evidence supporting the link between immune system characteristics and both prematurity and autism. I then propose a causation process model of autism etiology and pathogenesis, in which both neurodevelopment and ongoing/prolonged neuro-inflammation are necessary pathogenetic component mechanisms. I suggest that the Mackie–Rothman sufficient component cause model discussed earlier can be interpreted as a mechanistic view of etiology and pathogenesis and can serve as an explanatory model for autism causal pathways. Finally, I compare mechanist and process views of etiological explanations.

Chapter 7: Combined Contribution. This chapter revolves around my paper "The etiological stance: Explaining illness occurrence" (Dammann 2017), which responds to a piece by Kelly, Kelly, and Russo, who argue "for an integration of social, behavioral, and biological factors in the explanation of pathogenesis" (Kelly, Kelly, and Russo 2014:308). I think that theirs is a small but important step in the right direction. I also think that terminological discrepancies need to be resolved, that the pathogenetic perspective should be replaced with an etiological one, that we need to reconsider whether the concept of a "lifeworld" is necessary (because it does not provide information on how biological, behavioral, and social mechanisms can be linked mechanistically), and that we should move from "mixed mechanisms" to the "combined contributions" of factors in etiological explanations of illness. Moreover, I offer a more detailed explication of what I consider *contributors* (inducers, modifiers, and mediators) and show how etiological explanations could become more comprehensive and perhaps even more useful when enhanced by the notion of combined contribution.

Chapter 8: Etiological Coherence. The last chapter is based on a paper on Hill's viewpoints (i.e., heuristics for causal reasoning in epidemiology) (Dammann 2018). It suggests that explanatory coherentist theories, such as that offered by Ted Poston (Poston 2014), would provide an excellent starting point for formal epistemology projects designed to support causal decision-making in the health sciences. I added more detail as to why I think that Hill's heuristics *are* an explanatory coherentist view of causal explanation in epidemiology. I also propose examples of how future research could build on my analysis and discussion in this book.

2

A MULTIDISCIPLINARY PROBLEM

More than two decades' worth of dinner party conversations have taught me that most consumers of health information tend to think that epidemiology is all about epidemics. While this is indeed what some epidemiologists do, most specialize in the collection and analysis of data about the occurrence of health phenomena that are not related to infections. Some are interested in *descriptive* information about occurrence patterns of illness. Others are *analytical* epidemiologists, with the goal to find causes by finding risk factors[1] via group comparisons.[2] They compare groups with certain risk factors to groups without those same risk factors. If the groups differ by just one risk factor *ceteris paribus*, it is assumed that outcome differences in these two groups are *due to* the risk factor.

Despite their success over the past century or so, epidemiologists still ruminate the question of what kind of evidence they need to be fully justified in moving from mere observed association to causal claim. I began thinking about the link between illness occurrence research in epidemiology and philosophical aspects of causation in the 1990s. Almost two decades later, the paper "Perinatal brain damage causation" was published. In that paper, my colleague Alan Leviton and I took the position that

> the more of the following criteria are fulfilled, the stronger the support for the contention that some risk factor for PBD (perinatal brain damage) might be a "causal" factor:
>
> - The factor precedes PBD;
> - The factor can produce PBD in the experimental setting;
> - It is (statistically) associated with PBD in (well-powered) observational studies; and
> - Its absence from populations reduces the prevalence of PBD compared to populations with the factor present, for example in clinical trials. (Dammann and Leviton 2007:286)

Since the publication of this paper, I have come to see that those four bullet points are by no means hard-and-fast criteria for causation. Instead, they are what epidemiologist Sir Austin Bradford Hill (1897–1991) called "viewpoints" in his classic paper on causal inference in epidemiology.[3] In this book, Hill's proposal will play a major role in an explanatory coherentist framework for etiological explanations.

2.1 EPIDEMIOLOGY: FINDING CAUSES OF ILLNESS

Modern epidemiology is "the study of the distribution and determinants of disease frequency in human populations" (Rothman et al. 2008b:32). It is one of the foundations of the health sciences in that it provides the methods to gather knowledge about constellations of candidate causes of illness, based on detailed observations in populations.[4] Since the 1940s and 1950s, "modern" epidemiology has developed from mainly infectious disease-oriented research into health risk research, broadly construed. Today, epidemiological research encompasses both population-based and clinical research, designed to elucidate occurrence patterns of health phenomena in so-called *observational studies*, as well as information about intervention effectiveness in so-called *clinical trials*. The intention is to help us understand the etiology of disease, improve treatment strategies, and predict the outcome of disease. Epidemiology includes multiple subspecialties defined by exposure (environmental, occupational, nutritional epidemiology, among others), by outcome (e.g., cancer epidemiology and neuroepidemiology), by population (e.g., pediatric and perinatal epidemiology), or by scientific perspective (e.g., molecular, genetic, and genomic epidemiology).

The major variables in epidemiology are time, space, and people characteristics. The first issue here is estimation of disease frequency to estimate the disease burden in populations. Are there disease occurrence patterns in time (e.g., seasonal peaks) or space (e.g., outbreaks) that help us understand the occurrence of the disease under investigation? What does it tell us if a disease occurs mainly in the spring but not so often in the fall? What can we learn from the frequent claim that multiple sclerosis occurs more often at a distance from the equator, rather than closer to it? How about the people involved? Are distinct groups of individuals at particularly high risk? The overarching principle in this area of investigation is to learn from disease occurrence patterns about etiology, the natural history of illness, so that targeted medical and public health interventions can be designed.

The two main causal questions in epidemiology are "What is a cause and how do we know one?" (Susser 1991). Finding an answer to these two questions is at the epicenter of epidemiological theory, simply because finding causes of illness is the declared goal of epidemiological research. Here are a few examples of how epidemiologists put it, although I see a caveat in each one:

> Epidemiology, therefore, is about measuring health, identifying the causes of ill-health and intervening to improve health. (Webb and Bain 2011:2)

The caveat here is that intervention is the job of nurses, physicians, public health officials, *inter alia*, not of epidemiologists.

> Its scope covers the description of disease patterns, the search for causes of disease, and practical applications related to disease surveillance, prevention, and control. (Oleckno 2008:1)

I would agree with this definition if "applications covered" does not include intervention itself. Suggestions for targets for interventions indeed come from epidemiology, but the interventions themselves come from health-care providers.

What are the specific objectives of epidemiology? First, to identify the *etiology* or *cause* of a disease and the relevant risk factors. (Gordis 2014:2)

This definition confuses the concepts mentioned. In my view, *risk factors* are candidate causes, and *etiology* consists of two things: causes and pathogenesis.

2.2 TERMINOLOGY

What follows are preliminary definitions of terms I will use frequently in this book. *Illness* is any disease, disorder, or defect that affects an individual's well-being and requires or receives medical attention. *Etiology* is the natural history of illness occurrence, including initial causes and subsequent pathogenetic and disease mechanisms. *Pathogenesis* is the biological process that connects causes with the onset of illness. *Exposures* are external risk factors, such as sunlight, cigarette smoke, or pesticides, that are capable of initiating the pathogenetic mechanism (represented by the black box in Figure 2.1). Multiple exposures can co-occur, or occur in sequence, and interact in initiating and maintaining pathogenesis. *Outcomes* are clinical signs or symptoms that qualify as markers of disease. As with exposures, patterns of characteristics define the outcome. The *etiological process* includes exposure and outcome as beginning and endpoint, as well as the pathogenetic mechanism(s) in between.[5]

The distinction between causes and pathogenesis of illness is marked by an important feature: their elucidation requires two very different approaches that are provided by two scientific fields, epidemiology and basic science. Epidemiologists study the occurrence of health phenomena by gathering data in populations and report their results as aggregate data, trying to single out risk factors they can suggest to their colleagues in public health as targets for intervention. Laboratory-based health scientists gain their knowledge by using experimental tools, their focus being on the biological mechanisms at the cellular and tissue microlevel. Comprehensive

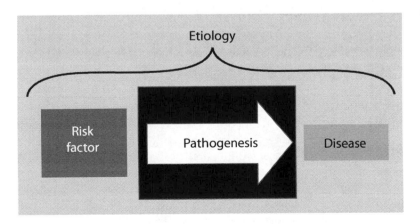

Figure 2.1 Etiology is the relationship between risk factor and disease. It includes the pathogenesis of illness, the biological mechanism that links risk factor and disease.

knowledge about the etiology of illness can be generated only if results from both fields are integrated.

The terms *etiology* and *pathogenesis* thus denote two very different but related notions. In their classic 1970 textbook *Epidemiology: Principles and Methods*, MacMahon and Pugh describe the notion of disease *etiology* as a two-part sequence. The first part is characterized by causal events prior to the initial somatic response that can be seen as the onset of disease in the individual. The second part is represented by "mechanisms within the body leading from the initial response to the characteristic manifestations of the disease."[6]

In this book, the disease is included as part of the pathogenesis, and thus of etiology, because some "characteristic manifestations of the disease" may occur long after the disease has become clinically manifest. Consider, for example, progressive disorders such as Parkinson's disease, a slowly progressing neurological condition with loss of muscle control and impaired movement. In many patients, the earliest signs of Parkinson's disease include tremor, a rhythmic shaking of the fingers, then hands, then arms. However, the pathogenetic process, a lack of the neurotransmitter dopamine that results from the destruction of dopamine-producing nerve cells in the brain, continues, and signs and symptoms often become worse, including more severe movement difficulties, sleep problems, cognitive and sensory difficulties, and depression. This changing clinical picture of Parkinson's disease after first clinical onset is relevant to its causal story and, therefore, the entire *disease process* should be considered part of its pathogenesis.

This *pathogenetic process* consists of a series of intra-individual biological changes, sometimes described as four stages between exposure and clinical disease (internal dose, biologically effective dose, early biological effect, and altered structure/ function) that provide the biological link between exposure and outcome (Schulte and Perera 1993). Although MacMahon and Pugh did not use the term *pathogenesis*, Khoury probably does not misquote them when they state that "disease is viewed as the result of a chain of events that comprise an intricate 'web' of external causal events and internal pathogenetic mechanisms" (Khoury 1993:12). In an ideal world, interventions on causal events will help prevent illness, while interventions on pathogenetic mechanisms will help treat illness once it has begun.

2.3 ETIOLOGY: TELLING THE STORY OF ILLNESS OCCURRENCE

Decades of successful epidemiological contributions to public health support these notions. Contributions come in the form of *etiological stories*, like the one on sitting as the new smoking. For example, regular exercise is associated with a reduced risk for a whole host of chronic diseases including heart disease, cancer, depression, and others. Many of these diseases are also associated with obesity and inflammation. An active lifestyle leads to both reduction in body fat and a less vigorous inflammatory response. Thus, both fat reduction and anti-inflammation are candidate mechanisms[7] for how exercise reduces the risk for those chronic diseases. The preventive intervention (exercise) is widely promoted with known success, although the mechanisms are still under investigation (Gleeson et al. 2011).

The causal role of smoking in lung cancer is still a matter of debate, although we have *very* strong evidence that smoking cessation reduces the incidence of lung disease. At least in part, the success of causation deniers is rooted in the fact that the pathogenetic mechanism is not yet fully understood and, perhaps, never will be. In a recent review article on the topic, the author states that

> It is the complexity of tobacco carcinogenesis due to the presence of multiple carcinogens and toxicants however which continues to challenge investigators to identify specific mechanisms that fully explain the ways in which smoking causes lung cancer. (Hecht 2012:2724)

The successes of epidemiology-based intervention programs in public health and health promotion are evidence in support of the notion that, at least sometimes, *we do not need mechanistic inference.* Instead, we need useful causal information that helps us tell useful etiological stories. Perhaps the epidemiologists' *textbook goal*, to identify the causes of illness, is only part of a more comprehensive de facto *goal*, that is, to help explain illness occurrence by contributing to etiological explanations. To do this, epidemiologists need to explicate the two-phase etiological process, which includes the *initiation* of the disease process by exposure to risk factors (a.k.a., candidate causes) and the *propagation* of the disease process via pathogenetic pathways.

Identifying the causes of illness (i.e., causal risk factors) is of interest for public health interventionists because the assumption is that illness can be prevented by eliminating such factors from populations. In this context, causes of illness are all factors that – if blocked from acting on individuals – are associated with a robust reduction in illness occurrence. In order to intervene medically, however, knowledge about the biological process from causation (initiation) to clinical disease is needed. This is the pathomechanism of disease, which is in the purview of medical bioscientists. Causal and pathogenetic stories of illness occurrence are sometimes told separately as the stories of illness causation and pathogenesis, respectively. In this view, etiology is the causal story *plus* the pathogenetic story that tells us about biological mechanisms in the body that occur in response to the causes.

In a different view, both are not considered separately but as two parts of the same concept:

> The etiology of a disease may be thought of as having a sequence consisting of two parts: (1) causal events occurring prior to some initial bodily response, and (2) mechanisms within the body leading from the initial response to the characteristic manifestations of the disease. (MacMahon and Pugh 1970:26)

This is what I have called the *etiological stance.*[8] I think that fast and successful progress in combating illness is more likely if epidemiologists are lumpers, not splitters, of causal and pathogenetic aspects of illness. However, telling overarching etiological stories requires taking an interdisciplinary perspective. This, in turn, requires epidemiologists to think deeply about how the causes they identify make sense as initiators of pathogenetic processes, and laboratory scientists to think deeply about whether the pathogenetic processes they study in the lab actually reflect the link between exposure-outcome constellations "out there." In essence, comprehensive etiological explanations require mutual interest and dialogue between epidemiologists and basic scientists, while isolated work may lead to situations in which successful development of helpful interventions becomes unlikely.

One prominent example from my own work is the etiology of what is sometimes called hypoxic-ischemic encephalopathy in preterm newborns. The attribute of "hypoxic-ischemic" (i.e., lack of oxygen and blood flow in the baby's brain) is based solely on experimental evidence that shows that hypoxia-ischemia *can* create brain damage in experimental animals, while we have no epidemiological evidence that hypoxia-ischemia actually *is* the (or at least one) cause of this kind of encephalopathy (Gilles et al. 2017).

This book has evolved from my recognition that questions about causation and causal inference asked by epidemiologists are closely linked to the kind of questions asked by classic philosophers of causation, including Hume, Mill, and Mackie; by philosophers of explanation, including Lewis, Salmon, Hempel, and Lipton; and by philosophers of medicine, such as Broadbent and Solomon. The current philosophy of science can be aligned in interesting ways with both the *textbook goals* of epidemiology, that is, identification and quantification of causal relationships, and also with its de facto goals, that is, contributing to useful etiological explanations for illness occurrence.

In what follows, I dig a bit deeper into the two main causal questions in epidemiology as mentioned earlier: what is a cause, and how do we know one? Philosophically speaking, the first is a metaphysical question (Section 2.4), and the second is an epistemological one (Section 2.5).

2.4 EPIDEMIOLOGICAL METAPHYSICS: WHAT IS A CAUSE?

The search for causes for illness has a long history.[9] Until today, the discussion of causation and causal inference has been one of the most intriguing and long-standing in epidemiology. It is also one of the most vibrant topics debated in philosophy of science. However, some epidemiologists think that the field lacks a solid theoretical foundation. For example, the promotional text for Nancy Krieger's book includes the following statement:

> Epidemiology is often referred to as the science of public health. However, unlike other major sciences, its theoretical foundations are rarely articulated. While the idea of epidemiologic theory may seem dry and arcane, it is at its core about explaining the people's health. (Krieger 2011)

One main assumption in this book is that philosophy of science has a lot to offer to epidemiologists who struggle with metaphysical and epistemic aspects of causation. As such, my project is situated at the interdisciplinary intersection between epidemiology and philosophy in a new field called "philosophy of epidemiology" (Broadbent 2013).

A few courageous philosophers and epidemiologists have an ongoing discussion about causality and causal inference in epidemiology.[10] Still, we are far from having agreement on what constitutes a cause of illness. For the purpose of the present discussion, I adhere to the epidemiological definition of *cause* as

> an antecedent event, condition, or characteristic that was necessary for the occurrence of the disease at the moment it occurred, given that other conditions are fixed. (Rothman et al. 2008c:6)

Moreover, no attempt to identify "the" core meaning of illness causation has led to an agreed-upon method for causal inference based on epidemiological data. Who says there is only one kind of cause, hence only one way to define causation (Cartwright 2004)? Perhaps there are many kinds, too many to be unified into one reasonable framework for illness causation research. MacMahon and Pugh support the notion that the term *causation* appears to have "different meanings in different contexts" (MacMahon and Pugh 1970:17).

A look at the current literature confirms that epidemiologists have neither a comprehensive metaphysical account of illness causation nor a clear epistemological concept of causal inference. For example, Parascandola and Weed begin their oft-cited essay on epidemiological definitions of causation with the statement that it is unclear that epidemiologists have one "single shared concept" of causation (Parascandola and Weed 2001). Their literature review identifies no less than five different definitions of causation in epidemiology: production, necessity, sufficient-component causes, probabilistic cause, and counterfactual causes. It is obvious that these definitions are closely related to philosophical accounts of causation.[11]

Here is what Parascandola and Weed found in a nutshell. The production definition of causation in epidemiology is simply the notion that causes produce, affect, or alter their effects. The necessary or sufficient definition of causation in epidemiology is the same as in philosophy: an effect cannot occur without the necessary cause and will occur with the sufficient cause. The sufficient-component cause model is Rothman's model in which multiple different constellations of (necessary or unnecessary) component causes represent sufficient causal complexes.[12] Finally, the counterfactual definition is that a cause makes a difference in the outcome when it is present compared to the situation when it is absent.[13] Parascandola and Weed suggest that it is likely that some combination of these definitions might be the "best fit" for epidemiology. For example, they point out that Nancy Cartwright's definition (C causes E iff $P[E | C.Kj] > P[E | Kj]$ for all Kj) employs both probabilistic and counterfactual elements (Cartwright 2004). They conclude that

> a counterfactually-based probabilistic definition is more amenable to the quantitative tools of epidemiology, is consistent with both deterministic and probabilistic phenomena, and serves equally well for the acquisition and the application of scientific knowledge. (Parascandola and Weed 2001:905)

As cogent as this may sound to epidemiologists, this statement does not provide any insight beyond why certain philosophical concepts seem to be the "best fit" for what epidemiology actually does while others do not. The authors admit that "a definition is not itself a theory of causation."[14] Part of my motivation for this book is that providing a theory for etiological explanations might be more fruitful than providing a theory of causation because epidemiology is not simply a method to find causes of illness. Instead, epidemiology is a comprehensive explanatory framework to elucidate the story of illness occurrence.

2.4.1 The Mackie–Rothman model

Echoing John Stuart Mill (1806–1873), Ken Rothman suggested in 1976 in his seminal paper "Causes" that it always takes multiple causes for disease occurrence, and that necessary and sufficient causes should not be considered at the same explanatory level.[15] Each of the three "pies" in Figure 2.1 represents one possible constellation of causal factors that, together, are sufficient to cause the illness of interest. Each wedge or piece of pie represents a component cause, which is necessary only if it is a component of all possible sufficient causal constellations (wedge A in pies I, II, and III).[16] If a component cause is present only in some but not all sufficient causes, it is unnecessary. Only if all component causes of each possible sufficient causal complex are present does illness occur. Based on these specifications, Rothman offers the following definition:

> A cause is an act or event or a state of nature which initiates or permits, alone or in conjunction with other causes, a sequence of events resulting in an effect [...] all kinds of causal factors form a "causal complex," "causal web," or "web of causation" that contributes to the development of illness. Each single factor is neither necessary nor sufficient, for producing the disease state, but their combination and potentiation lead to the effect. (Rothman 1976:588)

Rothman specifies three different categories of causes: (1) sufficient causes represented by pies I, II, and III in Figure 2.1; (2) necessary component causes that are part of all known possible sufficient causes of a disease of interest (i.e., piece A in all pies); and (3) non-necessary component causes that are neither sufficient nor necessary (pieces B–U). Note that Rothman uses the term *cause* in two very different ways. The first (sufficient cause = whole pie) means a causal complex that consists of multiple components. The second (component cause = piece of pie) means just one such member of the sufficient causal complex. Thus, Rothman's sufficient pies can be thought of as *determining* the occurrence of illness. Those who wish to fix this problem (of determinism) can "simply think of the components as contributing together to the probability of the effect, rather than being sufficient for it" (Parascandola and Weed 2001:280).

Let me propose a different perspective. Let's consider each pie a *comprehensive etiological explanation*. Each of these includes the initiator (cause) of the pathogenetic process and the pathogenetic mechanism. In Figure 2.2, for example, B and O could represent two such causes, which alone or together can initiate the etiological process, which consists of the cause itself (B, O, or both), one or more pathomechanisms (C, D, E, ...), and other contributors,[17] depicted by combinations of all pieces C–U, except B and O. The necessary component A could represent a necessary background condition, such as neurodevelopment in the explanatory model of autism causation I proposed with Carmina Erdei (Erdei and Dammann 2014).[18]

The sufficient-component cause model stands in the tradition of the work of philosophers J. S. Mill (1806–1873) and J. L. Mackie (1917–1981), who had written

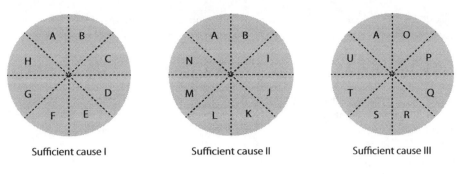

Sufficient cause I   Sufficient cause II   Sufficient cause III

Figure 2.2 The sufficient-component cause model of illness causation. (Based on Rothman, K. J. 1976. *Am J Epidemiol* 104:87–92.)

extensively about aspects of multicausality. Mill had discussed the idea that it is rarely one but often the joint effect of several antecedents that leads to an effect.[19] A few years before Rothman published his pies, South African epidemiologist Mervyn Susser (1921–2014) had also promoted "the logic of multiple causes" in the fourth chapter in his book *Causal Thinking in the Health Sciences* (Susser 1973). The multifactorial concept of illness causation holds that

> all kinds of causal factors form a "causal complex", "causal web" or "web of causation" that contributes to the development of illness. Each single factor is neither necessary nor sufficient, for producing the disease state,[20] but their combination and potentiation lead to the effect. (Dekkers and Rikkert 2006:280)

Perhaps Rothman was also inspired by J. L. Mackie (1917–1981), who published his idea of *insufficient but necessary part of an unnecessary but sufficient* (INUS) condition in book form (Mackie 1974). In pie lingo, the insufficient but necessary thing would be a piece of a pie, and the unnecessary but sufficient thing would be one of multiple possible whole pies.

The Mackie–Rothman INUS-Pie framework is the basis for a *top-down multilevel explanatory model of illness occurrence* for the biomedical sciences. The standard interpretation of the Mackie–Rothman model is that each complete pie depicts one of multiple *sufficient causes*. Another way is to let the complete pie represent a *sufficient etiological mechanism,* the instantiation of which is the etiological process that leads to the disease at hand. Granting the exposure of interest a spot among the pieces of the pie enables us to view the whole pie not just as an indicator of the fact that the causal complex is complete and the outcome occurs. It also enables us to view the complete pie as a causally sufficient constellation of risk factors (exposures, initiators) and (a sequence of) pathogenetic mechanisms that are jointly instantiated as an *etiological process,* which is responsible for illness occurrence. In this etiological interpretation of the model, what can be observed by epidemiologists is the exposure (the initiator of the pathogenetic mechanism) and the outcome (disease occurrence). In this sense, epidemiological observations are, technically speaking, *macro-etiological observations.*

At the *pathogenetic* level, the development of a disease is characterized by intrapersonal molecular and biochemical processes that lead to atypical body structure, function, or both. Each pathogenetic mechanism, depicted as one piece of the pie, is a blueprint for the instantiation as a pathogenetic process that contributes to the etiology of the disease under investigation. Since pathogenetic mechanisms, at least at the biological (cellular, molecular) level, cannot be observed in epidemiological studies, observations of pathogenetic processes are, technically speaking, *micro*-etiological observations.

For example, the initiating risk factor "prolonged exposure to ionizing radiation" is one pathogenetic process that, together with the background condition "aberrant DNA-breakage repair gene," leads to the pathogenetic process "DNA double-strand breakage," which in turn leads to the pathogenetic process "aberrant cell generation." Together with the necessary background condition "tissue growth," these factors form a sufficient etiological process that leads to skin cancer. Epidemiologists can observe the exposure to radiation as well as the presence of modifiers such as the DNA repair gene, and the occurrence of skin cancer. They cannot, however, elucidate details of the DNA breakage and abnormal cell growth processes; this work is left to wet bench scientists.

2.4.2 From pies to bicones

In the previous section, I have outlined the possibility of viewing each complete Mackie–Rothman pie as one distinct *sufficient etiological process* (SEP) that is sufficient to result in a certain illness. The pieces of each pie represent a combination of causes and pathogenetic mechanisms, such as causes, contributors, and background conditions identified by epidemiologists at the population level and biochemical pathophysiological processes studied by basic scientists in the wet lab. In this view, every SEP requires causal and pathogenetic components, some necessary, others unnecessary, to be complete and, thereby, to be sufficient.

In order to prevent illness, epidemiological work is geared toward finding preventable risk factors. In the INUS-Pie model, eliminating a necessary piece from a pie would eradicate the illness from the face of the earth (if there is only one possible pie/SEP for this disease). In medical history, infection with smallpox is the necessary component whose elimination made smallpox eradication possible. However, eliminating any unnecessary component would only reduce the likelihood of disease occurrence, because unnecessary components are (by definition) found in some but not all SEPs. Thus, knowledge of the components of the etiological process can help reduce the burden of illness in a variety of ways that are important in both medicine and public health.

During my early training as an epidemiologist, the Mackie–Rothman model always struck me as somewhat static, despite the fact that etiology is, of course, a process that develops along a timeline. What also struck me was the absence of the outcome in the visual depiction of the model's content. It seemed to me as if the model kept exposure and contributing factors and the outcome they contribute to somewhat artificially separate. Around that same time, I was reading Searle's 1984 Reith lectures, in which he describes the relationship between mind and brain as follows:

> Mental phenomena (...) are caused by processes going on in the brain (and) just are
> features of the brain. (Searle 1984:18,19)

My immediate intuition was that illness causation could be described similarly: diseases are caused by the exposure variables and at the same time are features of the system of exposure variables.[21] My way to depict this process idea of disease causation was to add a time dimension to the Mackie–Rothman sufficient-component model of illness causation (Figure 2.2), expanding the "pie" to be "nested bicones" (Figure 2.3). The exposure to a combination of risk factors (translucent outer bicone) starts at the beginning of the induction time[22] on the far left and leads to illness (in this figure, a particular disease; dark inner bicone). The dark ellipse in the center represents one of Rothman's pies, viewed from an angle.[23]

In the bicone model, a risk factor is conceptualized as both the cause of a disease and one of its characteristics, for example, smoking as both a cause and a characteristic of lung cancer. At the same time, a disease can be seen as both the effect of an exposure and as one of its characteristics, for example, lung cancer as an outcome and as a characteristic of smoking. According to this view, *risk factors and disease are two characteristics of the same process, that of illness etiology.*

This notion resonates with Mumford and Anjum's dispositionalist account of causation,[24] according to which "causes dispose towards their effects" (Mumford and Anjum 2011a:19) and "effects are brought about by powers manifesting themselves" (p. 7). Mumford and Anjum use the terms *powers* and *dispositions* exchangeably and mean "something that has possible manifestations, though it may nevertheless still exist unmanifested" (pp. 4–5).

My proposal that illness causation is *an etiological process* is accommodated by the dispositionalist view of causation as "a single unfolding process" (Mumford and Anjum 2011b:ix). Dispositionalist theories of causation are process theories, in which properties are gradually replaced: "causation is process-like in that one property (being solid, being cold) is gradually replaced by another (being dissolved, being warm) in a continuous alteration through intermediate properties (being partially

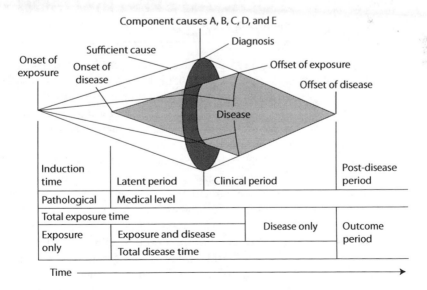

Figure 2.3 Extended Mackie–Rothman model of illness causation.

dissolved, being mild)" (Mumford and Anjum 2011b:124). Etiological explanations also take a process perspective, as outlined in Chapter 6. One way to put it would be to say that an etiological process occurs when an individual gradually transitions from being healthy to being clinically sick via a preclinical pathogenetic process.

Power philosophers also suggest that background conditions count as causes. They write that "[t]he distinction between causes and background conditions is not an ontologically grounded one, but rather a pragmatic or epistemological one. If all contribute to an effect, then they are causes of it" (Mumford and Anjum 2011a:33). This view, in turn, resonates well with my proposal in Chapter 6 to consider the combined effects of contributors to illness etiology. It also aligns well with the Mackie–Rothman model,[25] where each sufficient constellation of mutually accountable causal partners is depicted as one complete pie I, II, or III (Figure 2.2). Only when all components that belong to such sufficient cause are present is disease likely to occur. This notion of sufficient causal constellations (I would rather call them sufficient etiological constellations) as being less than deterministic has been proposed by Parascandola and Weed (2001). The view accommodates probabilistic views of causation as well as the dispositionalist view that a sufficient cause does not necessitate its effect but rather tends toward it.

In the remainder of this book, I take the following view of "illness causation," as broadly construed: Illness causation is a two-phase process that begins with (a) external initial triggers (risk factors, exposures) that initiate and/or maintain (b) internal pathogenetic processes (functions or dysfunctions) in the individual that (c) culminate in illness phenotypes (diseases). The *etiological process* is the entire process (a, b, c), from initial trigger to clinical disease. The *causation process* includes causes and pathogenesis (a, b), while the *disease process* includes pathogenesis and clinical disease (b, c).

2.5 EPIDEMIOLOGICAL EPISTEMOLOGY: CAUSAL INFERENCE

Epidemiologists approach the issue of causal inference by searching for risk factors that can be considered candidate causes. They conduct large-scale studies with human participants, measure exposures (such as smoking) and outcomes (such as cancer), and create multivariable mathematical models that yield an estimate of the relative risk (RR) for developing the outcome, which tells us, for example, how much more likely smokers are to develop cancer compared to nonsmokers.[26] Epidemiological theoreticians have developed an impressive methodological toolbox that includes methods for multivariable risk estimation, strategies to minimize bias, and techniques to adjust for confounding (Rothman, Greenland, and Lash 2008a). This research strategy has been tremendously successful. Across the globe, in rich as well as in developing countries, epidemiologists have helped prevent illness in populations. Control of infectious disease and vaccination programs, decline of cardiovascular death due to heart attack and stroke, fluoridation of drinking water, and recognition of tobacco smoke as a health hazard are only a few of the great achievements of public health in the twentieth century that can be attributed to successful epidemiological research (Centers for Disease Control and Prevention 1999, 2011).

2.5.1 Risk factors as candidate causes

In medicine, causal attribution has a long and colorful history. Vandenbroucke[27] refers to Anne Fagot-Largeault's thesis on causes of death, in which the author discusses the phenomenon that in medicine, causal inference is frequently performed by some kind of "detective-like-back-reasoning" from effects back to their putative causes.[28] Based only on case series, with no controls or confounder adjustments, causal powers are attributed to individual antecedents based on repeated observations and are then generalized without further ado. For some reason, Vandenbroucke writes, "modern medicine seems to escape at least in part – from today's dogmas that all our investigations and reasoning should be 'hypothetico-deductive'" (SII 16).[29]

Epidemiologists take such a hypothetico-deductive approach. Their goal is to discover factors that are associated with changes in disease occurrence. These factors are called *risk factors*, which may be risk reducers or risk increasers. In a second step, they distinguish statistical from causal association.

The concept is not novel. Consider this lengthy but illuminating quote from *On Airs, Waters, and Places*, in which Hippocrates offered a description of factors one should consider when looking at differences in health outcomes:

> Whoever wishes to investigate medicine properly, should proceed thus: in the first place to consider the seasons of the year, and what effects each of them produces for they are not at all alike, but differ much from themselves in regard to their changes. Then the winds, the hot and the cold, especially such as are common to all countries, and then such as are peculiar to each locality. We must also consider the qualities of the waters, for as they differ from one another in taste and weight, so also do they differ much in their qualities. In the same manner, when one comes into a city to which he is a stranger, he ought to consider its situation, how it lies as to the winds and the rising of the sun; for its influence is not the same whether it lies to the north or the south, to the rising or to the setting sun. These things one ought to consider most attentively, and concerning the waters which the inhabitants use, whether they be marshy and soft, or hard, and running from elevated and rocky situations, and then if saltish and unfit for cooking; and the ground, whether it be naked and deficient in water, or wooded and well watered, and whether it lies in a hollow, confined situation, or is elevated and cold; and the mode in which the inhabitants live, and what are their pursuits, whether they are fond of drinking and eating to excess, and given to indolence, or are fond of exercise and labor, and not given to excess in eating and drinking.[30]

This is a description of what modern epidemiologists call *risk factors*, although it is unlikely that Hippocrates had this concept in mind when he wrote this passage centuries before the Common Era. He suggested that the health status of a person or population is affected by winds and waters, nutrition, and exercise, long before modern epidemiology confirmed the notion.

Risk factors are what most of those who discuss illness causation mean when they talk about causes of illness. In a perfect world, one without error, bias, confounding, and residual mischief, risk factors *are* chance-of-outcome-changing causes. Thus, one way to tell the story of disease occurrence, the etiological story of the disease, is to give a list of its causes, to describe the natural history of illness in the language of risk, risk factors, and RR. Another way is to give a detailed description of the biochemical process, the pathogenetic mechanism that unfolds subsequent to its causal initiation.

The *risk factor* concept has been vigorously debated. The late Petr Skrabanek (1940–1994) considered risk factor epidemiology to be equivalent to a "black box" approach, where "an association (between exposure and disease), by itself a fortuitous finding, is thus converted, by logical sleight-of-hand, into a causal link" (Skrabanek 1994:553). He postulated that "the aim of science is to find universal laws governing the world around us and within us; it is about dismantling the 'black box'" and went on to suggest that "black box epidemiology is not science."[31] According to one reader's interpretation of Skrabanek's commentary, one of the weaknesses of black box epidemiology is that the causal model under investigation is not only unknown but "may even be considered irrelevant" (Smith 2001:327). The reader goes on to suggest that epidemiology and basic science are "feeding off each other [and] can contribute in a fundamental way to our understanding of disease." This is my point exactly, because both epidemiology and basic science contribute to the generation of comprehensive etiological explanations.

This is not a new idea. Less radical visions have been published as early as in 1959, when Yerushalmy and Palmer proposed to move from etiology concepts in infectious diseases to etiology in chronic diseases (Yerushalmy and Palmer 1959:39). They suggested three points they hoped might serve "as a first approach toward the development of acceptable guideposts for the implication of a characteristic as an etiologic factor in chronic disease": (1) increased presence of the characteristic in cases compared to controls, (2) increased incidence of disease in persons with the characteristic than in those without, and (3) absence (or at least small likelihood) of third factors that explain the association between the characteristic and the disease (exclusion of confounding factors). Lilienfeld suggested additional ways to "increase the likelihood of the causal hypothesis," that is, experiments in humans and laboratory animals and further epidemiologic research into the consistency of the findings (Lilienfeld 1959:46). Lilienfeld mentions further that problems with inferences from the animal to the human system "may be a minor problem if all types of data ... fit together in a consistent pattern." My view that multiple different studies offered by independent research groups are needed to support a causal hypothesis[32] stands in the Lilienfeldian tradition. Until we give up our dualist hope that we will at some point be able to extract causation from data, we should continue the scientific discourse based on results from experiments and observations, conducted in the laboratory and in epidemiologic studies.

Risk research needs to integrate benchwork and epidemiology, molecular biology, and social science. The endeavor is a social project.[33] Causal inference is a social activity being advanced by epidemiologists, philosophers, and bench scientists. However, the platforms of scientific discourse, conferences, and journals are very rarely interdisciplinary. To the contrary, they are often very specialized with regard to the scientific topic and methods applied. Although interdisciplinarity is generally considered helpful, it is not practiced widely or effectively. To replace "we cannot identify causation from data" with "we have agreed on an etiological explanation based on observation, experiment, and discourse" would provide us with a more hopeful and interesting outlook for future research.

If we can identify preventable risk factors, and if targeting these risk factors with interventions actually helps reduce the population burden of illness, isn't one justified to conclude that epidemiologists are capable of identifying *causes* of illness? Don't we all know intuitively how to draw correct causal inferences from observed data? Epidemiologists Miguel Hernán and Jamie Robins think that

> as a human being, you have already mastered the fundamental concepts of causal inference. You certainly know what a causal effect is; you clearly understand the difference between association and causation; and you have used this knowledge constantly throughout your life. In fact, had you not understood these causal concepts, you would have not survived long enough to read this chapter – or even to learn to read. As a toddler you would have jumped right into the swimming pool after observing that those who did so were later able to reach the jam jar. As a teenager, you would have skied down the most dangerous slopes after observing that those who did so were more likely to win the next ski race. As a parent, you would have refused to give antibiotics to your sick child after observing that those children who took their medicines were less likely to be playing in the park the next day.[34]

Such commonsensical concepts of causal knowledge acquisition may explain how we learn that flipping a light switch is a great strategy to illuminate the room at night. However, I think that this "electrical-circuit-view" of causation and causal learning is not a good metaphor for etiological reasoning in the health sciences. First, the scenario depends on learning by intervention (switching the switch). In the health sciences, only wet bench experiments and randomized clinical trials rely on intervention as a contributor to the generation of evidence in support of causal notions. The vast majority of epidemiological research is, however, observational in nature, where intervention and manipulation play no role whatsoever. Second, the human body is not a simple electric circuit, and it does not function that way. Instead, it is a highly complex biological organism. This complexity, the sheer number of biochemical reactions and physical-mechanical processes, and their biological interactions preclude simplistic deterministic causal inference. Third, the biochemical processes include elements that explain the transmission of information from one level (e.g., antigens as molecular structures) to another (e.g., cell-surface receptor activation).[35] The transmission of information across levels of biological systems is a ubiquitous characteristic of biological causation and, therefore, our understanding of etiological processes. Fourth, feedback loops are an important feature of biological phenomena in the human body; they are so important that at least one philosopher suggests to amend current definitions of "mechanism" to reflect this circular feature of biological mechanistic explanations (Bechtel 2011). Finally, the functions of all those causal and pathogenetic processes are extremely diverse. For example, signal transmission in the brain, in the muscular system, or in the liver is custom-tailored to the respective cellular and tissue environment. While some of these processes may share functional similarities, explaining their differences will require qualitatively different ways to provide causal, pathogenetic, and eventually etiological explanations.

The current literature on causation and causal inference in epidemiology comprises two clusters of publications: one written by epidemiologists and one by philosophers. I provide brief introductions to both in the next two sections.

2.5.2 The epidemiological perspective

Over the past decades, a large number of publications in epidemiological journals have addressed the following questions: what are causes (in epidemiology), and how can we find them (using epidemiological methods)?[36] The consensus seems to be that criteria cannot be used to establish causal claims with certainty.[37] Some hold that it is *impossible* to assert the presence of a causal relationship with certainty, because it is an inference about an exposure-outcome (i.e., risk factor–illness) relation and cannot be observed.[38] Cancer epidemiologist Douglas Weed offered a concise summary of three fundamental problems that, taken together, explain why causal hypotheses can never be established with certainty.[39] First, the "fundamental problem of causal inference" is that we cannot observe in the same individual both the effect of a cause and the noneffect in its absence. Second, the "fundamental problem of causal logic" is that scientific evidence can never determine whether the causal hypothesis, alternative hypotheses, or chance determined the particular situation. Third, the "fundamental problem of causation" is that causation is not observable; we see only our evidence, not causation itself. In sum, Weed thinks that causation exists, but that

> causation cannot be seen. Causation cannot be proven ... Nor can causation be made certain. It is, at best, an expert's judgment, at worst, an expert's guess.[40]

If it is true that causation can never be established from association (Pearson 1900; Skrabanek 1994), how can we ever identify it? It seems that we are stuck in something like the Plato-Cartesian dualism of surface data associations versus underlying causal structure. In fact, how much of our shying away from causal statements is because we *define* association and causation as being indistinguishable by simple observation? If we *define* observed data as insufficient for causal inference, we cannot identify causation from observed data by definition.

2.5.2.1 Bradford Hill's viewpoints

One main technique for causal inference described in epidemiology textbooks is based on a paper published in the mid-1960s (Hill 1965). The author, Sir Austin Bradford Hill, was an epidemiologist who was deeply involved, together with his colleague Sir Richard Doll, in the research that led to the now widely accepted notion that tobacco smoking causes lung cancer.[41] Hill's paper is the written version of the president's address he gave in 1964, shortly after the founding of a new Section of Occupational Medicine of the Royal Society of Medicine. The paper is a summary of views about causation published by the Surgeon General's advisory committee on smoking and lung cancer (U.S. Surgeon General's Advisory Committee on Smoking and Health 1964), generated over multiple years of discussion and a "series of formative events and exchanges among U.S. experts who created the guidelines used by the U.S. advisory committee" (Blackburn and Labarthe 2012:1071). Hill outlined his perspective on characteristics of observational epidemiological research results (which he called "viewpoints") that may help in making the decision whether an observed association between exposure and outcome is causal. These aspects of associations are

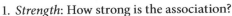

1. *Strength*: How strong is the association?
2. *Consistency*: Does the association fit with findings by others under different circumstances?
3. *Specificity*: Is the association present between specific risk factors and specific outcomes?
4. *Temporality*: What is the cause, and what is the effect?
5. *Biological gradient*: Does the outcome risk increase with increasing exposure levels?
6. *Plausibility*: Is the association biologically plausible?
7. *Coherence*: Is the association in keeping with known biological facts and characteristics of the disease's natural history?
8. *Experiment:* Does intervention reduce disease occurrence?
9. *Analogy:* Do we have evidence from associations between similar risk factors and similar outcomes?

Hill was extremely careful to avoid deterministic notions, always making sure the reader understands that these characteristics are not *necessary* for causal inference, just aspects to consider before jumping from observed association to inferred causation. In epidemiology and the health sciences, Hill's viewpoints serve as one standard model for causal inference. Ironically, the scientific and philosophical consensus is that they cannot be used as criteria for illness causation.[42]

What is the value of Hill's viewpoints if they cannot serve as criteria? While some degrade Hill's viewpoints to the level of a "traditional" method in contrast to their "modern" approach,[43] others think of Hill's approach as the *sui generis* method for causal inference in epidemiology (Morabia 2013). In this book, Hill's viewpoints (and, by extension, mine) are taken to be explanatory virtues in a coherentist framework of causal explanation (Dammann 2018). I refer mainly to Poston's recent defense of explanatory coherentism (Poston 2014). According to his theory,

> explanationism is a general view about epistemic justification. The justificatory status of one's beliefs is determined by the explanatory merits of one's system of beliefs (…) an epistemological defense of explanationism should indicate which virtues are relevant for epistemic justification. (Poston 2014:80)

The bottom line of my proposal is that each one of Hill's characteristics can be viewed as an explanatory virtue on an explanatory coherentist framework for etiological explanation.[44] My intention is to get to a more rigorous understanding of what we mean when we talk about Hill's viewpoints, so we can place them within a theoretical framework about the nature of evidence for causation, and about the nature of causal inference.

Bradford Hill came from the environmental/occupational epidemiology perspective; he was interested in relationships between exposures (work conditions that represent risk factors) and outcomes (illness). Therefore, he offered an informal framework to "detect relationships between sickness, injury, and conditions of work" (Hill 1965:295).

2.5.2.2 Potential outcomes

Perhaps the most prolific epidemiologist with a primary interest in causation and causal inference is Miguel Hernán (Hernán 2004; Hernan and Robins 2006a; Hernan et al. 2002), whose definition of a causal effect (for an individual) is that treatment T has a causal effect on outcome O (in that individual) if O looks different depending on whether treatment T is administered to that same individual or not (Hernan and Robins forthcoming).

This counterfactual concept of "potential outcomes" is currently gaining traction in the public health literature (Glass et al. 2013). The main philosophical problem with the potential outcomes approach is that it is epistemologically empty. We cannot observe all potential outcomes, only the one that occurs. (This is Weed's "fundamental problem of causal inference.") Thus, potential outcomers are stuck where we all are between a rock and the problem of induction. It is *not* my goal to criticize the potential outcomes approach in this book. I do not think that such a critique would improve my general argument, because the potential outcomes approach is mainly a quantitative one that *presupposes* causal knowledge instead of generating it. In his book, *Explanation in Causal Inference*, Tyler VanderWeele writes that the potential outcomes framework

> provides formal criteria concerning when we can draw such conclusions about causation from empirical data; in other words for the assumptions that need to be made, or are sufficient, to move from conclusions about association to conclusions about causation. (VanderWeele 2015:5)

However, it is difficult to identify any such set of criteria anywhere in the potential outcomes literature. Perhaps the most comprehensive discussion of the POA's problems so far was sparked by a paper by Vandenbroucke, Broadbent, and Pearce in the *International Journal of Epidemiology* (Vandenbroucke, Broadbent, and Pearce 2016). In that paper, and in their response to subsequent commentaries, the authors offer a comprehensive analysis of the POA and a restricted version of it (RPOA). They specify four characteristics of what they call the "standard version" of the POA as follows:

> i. Counterfactual dependence of E on C is not necessary for C to cause E, but it is sufficient (POA's Basic Metaphysical Stance).
>
> ii. Sufficient evidential conditions currently exist for attributing the counterfactual dependence of E on C, but necessary conditions currently do not; the POA identifies some (but not all) of these sufficient conditions (POA's Basic Epistemological Stance).
>
> iii. Causal inference includes two distinct aspects: causal identification, in which the truth value of a claim of the form "C causes E" is determined; and quantitative causal estimation, in which a numerical value *n* is estimated for a claim of the form "C has *n* effect on E" (the Identification/Estimation Distinction).
>
> iv. Adequately well-defined counterfactual contrasts are necessary for giving meaning to quantitative estimates of causal effect (POA's Semantic Stance on Estimation). (Broadbent, Vandenbroucke, and Pearce 2016:1841)

The RPOA, according to Broadbent and colleagues, is characterized by one additional feature:

v. Counterfactual contrasts are adequately well-defined if and only if we can specify a corresponding adequately well-defined intervention on the putative cause, by which the counterfactual contrast would be (or would have been) brought about (RPOA's Restriction to Interventions). (Broadbent, Vandenbroucke, and Pearce 2016:1842)

I will not offer a comprehensive critique of the POA/RPOA in this book but refer to it and its explanatory weaknesses at multiple points in my discussion.

2.6 THE PHILOSOPHERS' PERSPECTIVE

The first book on *Health, Disease, and Causal Explanations in Medicine* came from Scandinavia (Nordenfelt and Lindahl 1984) and contained a collection of papers presented at a meeting in 1982. Among these, two[45] explicitly address criteria (Ahlbom 1984) and models of causation in epidemiology (Norell 1984).[46] Paul Thagard's *How Scientists Explain Disease* (1999) recounts the discovery process of *Helicobacter pylori* as an infectious agent that contributes to peptic ulcer causation. The book focuses on causal explanation, not inference. Thagard concludes that "science is a complex psychological, social, and physical system" and is characterized by "distributed computation," of which the scientific community is the underlying system (Thagard 1999:220). In 2003, K. Codell Carter published his case studies in the history of disease causation (Carter 2003). The book provides a collection of accounts of several theories of disease, including bacterial, viral, protozoal, ideational, and nutritional theories, mainly based on historical descriptions of discovery processes in the nineteenth century. In his "final thoughts," Carter asks "what, if anything, can we expect of future causal thinking in medicine?" (Carter 2003:200) and quotes Stehbens (Stehbens 1992), who, according to Carter, finds contemporary epidemiological concepts of causation imprecise and suggests paying attention to Aristotle, Spinoza, Hume, Mill, and Russell. As opposed to Stehbens, however, Carter thinks that "dead philosophers are in no position to advise epidemiologists about how to talk" (Carter 2003:202).

Two recent collections of papers on causality in the sciences contain chapters on causation in the health sciences. One was edited by Federica Russo and Jon Williamson (2007a) with Phyllis Illari joining them on the other (Illari, Russo, and Williamson 2011). In volume 16 of the *Handbook of the Philosophy of Science* devoted to "Philosophy of Medicine" (Gifford 2011), Daniel Steel has a chapter on "Causal inference and medical experiments" that is at least partially relevant for this book in the context of experimental, but not observational, studies. Other chapters in that volume, for example, on theories and models in medicine and on patterns on medical discovery, bear on my discussion as well. The first monograph devoting sustained attention to this topic is Alex Broadbent's *Philosophy of Epidemiology* (Broadbent 2013).

Phyllis Illari and Federica Russo advocate for a causal mosaicism, of integration across the sciences and philosophy; across types of causing, concepts of causation, types of inferences, sources of evidence; and across methods for causal inference (Illari and Russo 2014). They take a decidedly pragmatist approach in that they are action oriented and write that "causal notions have a role for different tasks" (Illari and Russo 2014:256) and that "different concepts help in building causal knowledge, in virtue of their usefulness for specific tasks."[47] In their last chapter, the authors describe how the scientific approach to the mosaic of lifetime exposures and their individual and joint health effects can be enriched by using their proposed causal mosaic. I share the authors' hope that many will use this approach to "think better about science."[48]

The philosophy of epidemiology is a rather young field, and the two main clusters of publications from epidemiology and philosophy reviewed in this and the previous section are waiting to be integrated. My goal in this book is to take a first step toward such integration.

2.7 "CAUSES OF EFFECTS" VERSUS "EFFECTS OF CAUSES"

Dawid, Faigman, and Fienberg discuss what they perceive as a disconnect in the context of scientific reasoning in legal contexts (Dawid, Faigman, and Fienberg 2014). Their discussion bears directly on the ways etiological explanation can be used in practice. The authors begin their discussion by pointing out that

> science studies individuals in order to make statements about populations, while the law considers populations in order to make statements about individuals.[49]

Let us call this the *population/person dyad*. In defense of the legal system, Dawid and coauthors acknowledge that

> courts are generally acquainted with the difficulties inherent in employing general scientific data to reach conclusions about specific cases.[50]

Let us call this the *type/token contrast*. The authors further stipulate that while judges and juries are looking for evidence in support of the *retrospective* conjecture that a certain effect was produced by certain causes (CoE), the science they rely on is primarily concerned with some kind of *prospective* conjecture that certain causes will yield certain effects (EoC). This is a bit like looking for the unknown parents of known children (CoE) versus looking for the unknown children of known parents (EoC). Let's call this the *EoC/CoE contrast*. Dawid et al. bring all three contrasts together, implying a parallel structure of sorts, by aligning science with population/type/EoC and legal with person/token/CoE (p. 361):

> [T]his produces a conundrum for the law and science connection. Science typically wishes to infer "the effects of causes (EoC), through experiments and observational studies, but legal fact finders need to infer "the causes of effects" (CoE). Legal fact finders cannot reasonably infer from general data alone that a particular effect is attributable to a known cause, yet they are ultimately charged with exactly this responsibility – of determining at some level of certainty what caused a particular effect. This question of how best to reason from group data to an individual case is pervasive in the courtroom use of science.

Dawid et al. conclude that "scientists could do much more in studying the matter of reasoning about the CoE."[51] I think that etiological explanation is one potential solution here. First, etiology is what connects causes and effects and can, thus, help in both EoC and CoE situations. Second, etiological explanations can explain both type and token events. Third, they work at both the population and person levels.

Before I offer support for these three related arguments (in Sections 2.7.2–2.7.4), I need to clarify (in Section 2.7.1) a common misunderstanding regarding the relationship between the population/person and type/token contrasts. In Section 2.7.5, I suggest that the cause-effect component of etiological explanation estimates the causal vigor by reference to the strength of the association between putative causes and their effects. The pathogenesis part of etiological explanation clarifies biologically what determines the causal vigor of a certain cause-effect relationship.

2.7.1 The population/type–person/token error

Dawid and coauthors write that

> courts are generally acquainted with the difficulties inherent in employing general scientific data to reach conclusions about specific cases

and

> … in medical causation cases, … they distinguish between "general causation" and "specific causation."[52]

Here, Dawid et al.'s distinctions become a bit murky. While the former quote ("courts are generally…") still seems to be about population data versus their application to a single person or event, the second quote ("in medical causation …") seems to refer to what is known in philosophy as *type* versus *token* contrast, which distinguishes between general law-like statements such as "smoking causes lung cancer" and particular situation-specific statements as in "his lung cancer was caused by his smoking." The type/token contrast is not identical to the contrast between causes of sickness in individuals and causes of the incidence rate of disease in populations.[53] Both type and token statements can be made with regard to both populations and persons. Consider the following statements: "the influenza virus causes epidemics in populations"; "the influenza virus causes a sickness with high fever in an infected person"; "in 1918, the influenza virus caused the deadliest pandemic in history"; and "last month, the influenza virus caused my brother to have a sickness with high fever."

Dawid and coauthors do not make it clear whether they think of the population/person contrast and the general/specific causation contrast as parallel but distinct contrasts, or as the same contrast. In other words, they are not entirely clear whether they think that the distinctions simply coexist or relate to each other, as in "science uses population approaches to generate knowledge about general causation" and "legal decisions require knowledge about specific causation in individuals." If the latter is the case, Dawid and coauthors commit what may be called the *population∼type/ person∼token error*. This error arises when it is assumed that talk about population data is the same as talk about a type-situation, and that talk about an individual is talk about a token situation. I do not think this is accurate, because "types are generally said to be abstract and unique; tokens are concrete particulars."[54] The distinction goes back to Peirce, who wrote that

> (In a manuscript or book) there will ordinarily be about twenty thes on a page, and of course they count as twenty words. In another sense of the word "word," however, there is but one word "the" in the English language; and it is impossible that this word should lie visibly on a page or be heard in any voice, for the reason that it is not a Single thing or Single event. It does not exist; it only determines things that do exist. Such a definitely significant Form, I propose to term a Type. A Single event which happens once and whose identity is limited to that one happening or a Single object or thing which is in some single place at any one instant of time, such event or thing being significant only as occurring just when and where it does, such as this or that word on a single line of a single page of a single copy of a book, I will venture to call a Token.[55]

Thus defined, both type and token situations can apply to both populations and persons. Take, for example, the measles in persons and in populations. If I refuse to have my child vaccinated, she is likely to get the measles upon exposure to the virus. My child is clearly a person, not a population. Should she really get the measles, this would be a single case in the sense of a token event. Now, the type-token dyad can play out in single individuals as follows. In the sense of a token event being the instantiation of type dispositions, any nonimmunized person is at risk of contracting the measles *in general*. If she does indeed develop the disease, however, her illness would qualify as a token event, an instantiation of the measles as a general disease concept. Along the same lines, a person is not an instantiation of a population but of the general concept of a person. Similarly, a population can be considered the instantiation of the concept of population, however defined.

Parallel to the occurrence of the measles in persons, measles occur in populations, not just in individual members of populations, but sometimes as what is called an "outbreak."[56] Any individual measles outbreak qualifies as a token event, an instantiation of the general concept of measles outbreaks. For example, we had six individual measles outbreaks in the United States in early 2019.[57] Each outbreak was monitored separately, and different actions to curb the epidemic were taken at local and regional levels. These six outbreaks are not the measles *type*; they are a group of instantiations of the concept of measles outbreaks. Instead, just as a group of persons can be defined as a population, a group of measles outbreaks can be defined (a bit awkwardly, I have to admit) as a population or group of measles outbreaks.

In sum, my sick child is an example of a token situation concerning a person, and one particular outbreak is a token situation concerning a population. Similarly, the concept of measles in individuals is a type situation that concerns persons, while the concept of measles outbreaks is a type situation that concerns populations.

2.7.2 Etiological explanation and the EoC/CoE dyad

Giving an etiological explanation is explaining illness occurrence by reference to its causes *and* pathomechanisms. In this section, I outline how etiological explanation

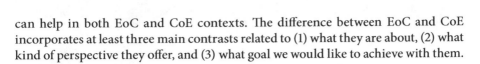

can help in both EoC and CoE contexts. The difference between EoC and CoE incorporates at least three main contrasts related to (1) what they are about, (2) what kind of perspective they offer, and (3) what goal we would like to achieve with them.

2.7.2.1 Subject

The first contrast is related to what EoC and CoE are *about*. Both EoC and CoE are ways of asking a question, but they obviously differ in what these questions are about. A search for EoC requires knowing the cause, so one can explore its potential effects. In contrast, a search for CoE requires knowing the effect, so one can explore its candidate causes. Clearly, the two perspectives are about two different *things*, causes versus effects, analyzed in relation to the respective other. If cause and effect are viewed as two *aspects* of the same thing, as in Mumford and Anjum's dispositionalist account of causal simultaneity, in which "the cause will be depicted as merging into and becoming the effect through a natural process,"[58] then the two perspectives are about one of the two aspects in light of the other. This brings us to the next contrast, that of time order of events in the causal process.

2.7.2.2 Process

One of the few aspects of causation that scientists, judges, and jury members, as well as philosophers agree on is that causation is about a sequence of events that *proceed* forward in time: causes first, effects later.[59] CoE questions require an assessment of evidence from past events, and they require taking a backward-looking perspective. The goal is to explain why some effect occurred *given the cause did occur*. In contrast, answering EoC questions requires the assessment of future events, taking a forward-looking perspective. It can be argued that the forward/backward contrast is *inherent* in the EoC and CoE concepts by definition, because both refer to the time order of events in a causal process.[60]

2.7.2.3 Goal

The third difference between EoC and CoE also pertains to their time order, but this time in relation to *what EoC and CoE data are needed for*. While EoC looks forward from cause to effect, CoE looks backward from effect to cause. In a sense, giving an EoC account is making a *prediction*, while giving a CoE account is giving an *explanation*. This view is captured in Miettinens'[61] analysis of "genera of causality in medicine." Miettinen (and his coauthor Karp) postulate the existence of "two genera of causality in medicine," that is, "etiogenetic and interventive"[62]:

> Ad-hoc knowing about etiogenetic causality – etiognosis, that is (cf. above) – is tantamount to having a causal explanation of an existent outcome (level of a morbidity, or presence of an illness); it thus inherently is retrospective from the vantage of an existent outcome. By contrast, ad-hoc knowing about interventive causality is a decision-relevant input into prognosis; it is knowing about the causal change in a future outcome resulting from an intervention, the adoption of which (notionally or actually) is a given; it is prospective from the vantage of the decision about adoption (or continuation) of the intervention.[63]

Behind the veil of stilted lingo Pearce calls "Miettinese" (Pearce 2012), one can see CoE being aligned with Miettinen and Karp's etiogenetic causality, and EoC aligned with their interventive causality. Although they entitle the pertinent section of their book "The two genera of causality in medicine," Miettinen and Karp do not write about etiogenetic and interventive causality as two different *kinds* of causality. Instead, they talk about "two types of *causal concern* in medicine,"[64] thereby opening the door for an interpretation of etiogenetic and interventive causality as two different ways of thinking about causality in medicine. These two foci of interest are clearly goal defined. In medicine as an intervention-focused profession, the former way of thinking is the focus for those who want to learn about the etiology of health phenomena and probably act on such knowledge, while the latter is the focus for those who are interested in the potential health outcomes of interventions.

2.7.3 Etiological explanation in populations and in persons

Etiological explanation is telling the story of illness occurrence at either the personal or the population level. At the personal level, the story is about the sequence of events, a detailed list of causal and pathomechanistic facts or events that occurred in a specific order and that culminated in the onset of illness. One example of such a sequence is the "chain of events" listed on death certificates; for example, death is the "onset of illness" to be explained, atherosclerotic coronary artery disease is the "underlying cause of death" that led to the "immediate cause of death" (rupture of myocardium) via inducing a thrombosis in the coronary artery with subsequent acute myocardial infarction. Taken as an etiological explanation, the sequence from thrombosis to myocardial rupture can be thought of as the pathomechanism that connects the underlying cause (atherosclerosis) with the death of the individual.

In populations, the "onset of illness" is marked as a change in the incidence[65] or prevalence[66] of a certain disease. These epidemiological measures give an estimate of the *disease burden* in a population, and they are, obviously, very different from the one we use in individuals. In explanatory terms, illness occurrence at the population level may have multiple possible etiological constellations, while there is usually only one in a person. Thus, etiological explanation at the population level is a meta-story, the story of all known stories of how a certain illness *can* occur and, thereby, contribute to an increasing incidence or prevalence of the disease in this population.[67]

2.7.4 Type and token etiology

Just as etiological explanation can refer to either an individual or to a population, it can be a token or a type explanation. If we explain why my aunt developed lung cancer, we can refer to *her* smoking behavior over decades as a cause, and to smoke-induced uptake of carcinogens with subsequent loss of normal lung cell growth *in her* lung as the pathomechanism. The type version of this explanation is when we refer to the same cause and mechanism for cancer development in anyone, *as a general rule*. In essence, both type and token etiological explanations refer to the same process depicted in Figure 2.4 but with reference to either the general concept or to one instance of it.

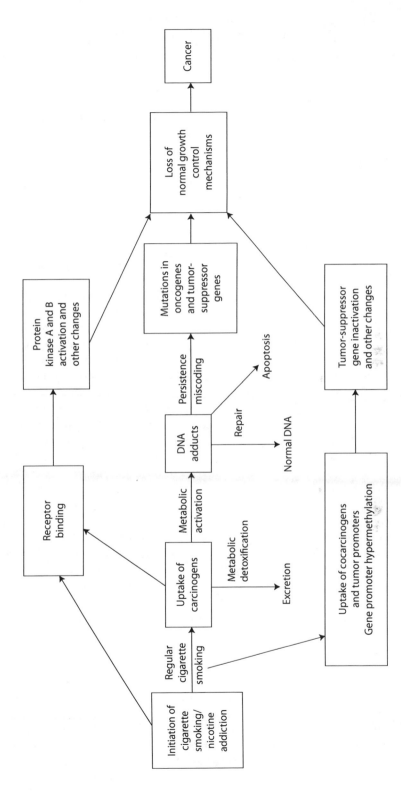

Figure 2.4 Etiological process from cigarette smoke exposure to cancer development. (From Office of the Surgeon General, How tobacco smoke causes disease: The biology and behavioral basis for smoking-attributable disease: A report of the Surgeon General, Washington, DC, 2010.)

2.7.5 Etiological explanations in science and the courtroom

Dawid and coauthors seem to view the EoC/forward and CoE/backward coupling as tied exclusively to the scientific and legal realms, respectively. They seem to propose that scientists produce data by looking forward, and juries apply those data backward. In other words, they hold something like "science produces evidence that justifies inference to EoC explanations that reason forward in time," while "judges and juries need evidence that justifies inference to CoE explanations that reason backward in time." Let's call this the direction-of-perspective contrast, which distinguishes between the perspective that takes a purported cause as the point of departure and observes its subsequent effects, and the perspective that takes a specific disease as the point of departure and observes its antecedent causes. Asking an EoC question is asking for a prediction, as in "What effect E will happen if cause C happens?" Asking a CoE question is probing the past: "What cause C might have been responsible for effect E to occur?"

The basic idea is that EoC and CoE are two very different things, because the questions asked have opposite directions in time. However, it is not the case that the EoC and CoE perspectives are taken exclusively in science and legal contexts, respectively. Nor do scientists and, for example, judges employ only EoC and CoE reasoning, respectively. In medicine, an EoC question is, "Will this pharmacological therapy help my patient?" An epidemiological EoC question is, "What is the long-term outcome after cerebral stent implantation?" Judges ask expert witnesses EoC questions when they ask, "Would the child have sustained brain injury had the obstetrician performed the cesarean section 20 minutes earlier?" A CoE question in medicine is, "What caused this patient's lung disease?" The epidemiologist wants to know "What are the causes of neonatal brain damage?" Similarly, the courtroom jury tries to answer the CoE question, "What caused this child's disability?"

Both scientific endeavor and legal procedures rely on a kind of discourse in their respective settings. For example, infectious disease scientists employ EoC reasoning when they set up experiments in which experimental animals are infected with a certain virus, and subsequent clinical effects are observed. Infectious disease epidemiologists employ CoE reasoning when they take serum samples from infected individuals and healthy controls, looking at the presence of viral antigen. Similarly, grand juries employ CoE reasoning when they want to identify what led to the murder, but they also employ EoC reasoning when they are considering how a known motive of the defendant may have led to the multiple possible cascades of events that ended with the death of the victim. In essence, both forward and backward reasoning is employed both in science and in legal cases.

In epidemiology, the direction-of-perspective contrast is of importance when considered in light of two fundamentally different types of epidemiological study, cohort and case-control studies. The former starts with study subjects sorted by exposure. (They either have the purportedly causal characteristic or they do not.) Then a wait ensues for a predefined study period (often years) to see whether the effect occurs or not. The latter starts with individuals classified by whether they have the disease (effect) under study or not, then looks back into the individuals' medical history, searching for evidence that they were exposed to the purported cause or not. However, it would be a mistake to consider only cohort studies as "EoC studies," and case-control studies only as "CoE studies," because there is yet another difference to consider. First, the terms *prospective* and *retrospective* can be used as descriptors of how the study was conducted in real time. When used in this sense, *prospective* means that while exposure status is already known when the study begins (the cause has occurred), the outcome (effect) has not yet occurred. Similarly, *retrospective* means that both exposure and outcome (cause and effect) have already occurred when the investigator launched the study. In this sense, both cohort and case-control studies can be either prospective or retrospective. Second, prospective and retrospective can be descriptors of which direction-of-perspective we obtain when looking at the data, either from exposure to outcome (from cause to effect) or from outcome back to exposure (from effect to cause).

2.7.6 Etiological explanation refers to causal vigor

Etiological explanations give a detailed account of the natural history of illness occurrence by reference to both causal and pathogenetic factors. Etiological explanation captures all three contrasts listed earlier.

First, etiological explanation is a narrative that covers causes, pathomechanisms, and clinical disease; how they relate to each other (Figures 3.1 and 6.1); as well as their relations to other explanatory factors (Figure 6.3). In the same etiological explanation, we cover both which effects "belong to" which causes (EoC) and which causes "belong to" which effects (CoE).

Second, etiological explanations describe the *process* that leads from initial causes via pathomechanisms to illness. Although this is an explanation that describes the etiology in a prospective fashion, the sequential relationship of events in this process is to a large part a sequence of regularities of the *if-then* kind.

Third, whether science is mainly about EoC and courtroom arguments mainly about CoE remains to be discussed in more detail. If we view the search for EoC as a desire to predict *what will happen if the cause occurs,* and the search for causes as an expression of a desire to be able to explain *why the effect occurred*, we are basically doing the same thing: we want to estimate the risk for an effect associated with a cause. *Risk* is, conceptually, a relationship between certain causes and certain diseases. Epidemiologists use a direction-neutral measure, the odds ratio (OR), to quantify the strength of the association between risk factor and disease. Viewed from the EoC perspective, the OR_{EoC} is estimated by dividing the outcome odds among the exposed by the outcome odds among the nonexposed. From the CoE perspective, the OR_{CoE} is estimated by dividing the exposure odds among those with the disease by the exposure odds among those without the disease (Figure 2.5).

Under certain conditions, either OR can be interpreted as quantifying the strength of the *disease risk* associated with a certain risk factor. More importantly, if data are tabulated in a fourfold table as the one in Figure 2.5, the values for OR_{EoC} and OR_{CoE} are numerically the same. Because ORs are unit-free and without direction in time or argument, and because they are being used as quantifiers of the strength of the association between potential causes (risk factors) on the one hand and effects

Effect

		Yes	No
Cause	Yes	a	b
	No	c	d

Odds Ratio (OR)	
CoE	a:c / b:d
EoC	a:b / c:d

Figure 2.5 Fourfold table listing the possible combinations of putative cause (risk factor) and effect (disease).

(diseases) on the other, they may also be indicators of the strength of the etiological explanation they are part of. In essence, I suggest that we have reason to assume that something like a *causal vigor* ties causes and effects together with a certain strength. In this view, ORs are quantifiers of the causal vigor that connects causes with effects.[68]

This point invalidates Dawid and coauthors' notion that "it is the relative risk RR, and not the OR, that is required for assessing CoE."[69] According to traditional epidemiological teaching, the RR can be calculated only in cohort studies, not in case-control studies, because the RR is calculated as the incidence rate of the outcome among the exposed divided by the incidence rate among the unexposed. The RR cannot be calculated in traditional case-control studies, because there is no such thing as incidence in a case-control setting, because the outcome has already occurred (in the cases) or not (in the controls), and nobody is waiting for further outcomes to occur. In traditional case-control studies, one can only estimate the RR by means of calculating the OR, which is derived from a fourfold table defined by exposure (+/−) and outcome (+/−) and is calculated as the cross-product ratio (number of exposed with outcome × number of nonexposed without outcome)/ (number of exposed without outcome × number of nonexposed with outcome). Therefore, the RR is a *directed* measure of RR, going from exposure to outcome, while the OR is *direction free*. For this reason, Dawid and coauthors consider the RR capable of supporting CoE claims apparently only because it is looking forward in time, while the OR's lack of direction disqualifies it from providing such support. However, this is not necessarily so, because in case-control studies that employ *incident* (not prevalent) cases, the case group builds up over time, and whoever does not develop the disease under investigation serves as a control. Such studies provide true risk estimates (considering relative exposure time), and the OR really does reflect the RR.

3 ETIOLOGICAL EXPLANATIONS

3.1 PHILOSOPHY OF EPIDEMIOLOGY

Alex Broadbent's *Philosophy of Epidemiology* is the first book-length treatment of epidemiological issues written by a philosopher. Among the many important points Broadbent raises, the following is particularly intriguing. In the synopsis of his book, he writes "causation is really only part of what we seek to measure and infer [...] what epidemiologists really seek to do is *explain,* and their practices are seen much more clearly when described as such" (Broadbent 2013:8). Along these lines, his main claim is that explanation is a more *useful* concept than causal inference if our goal is to understand measures of causal association and the nature of causal inference. In this chapter, the groundwork is laid for shifting the focus ever so slightly from causal inference to *etiological* explanation (EE).

What does Broadbent mean when he talks about explanation as a concept in this context? In order to explicate his position, Broadbent discusses the causal interpretation problem (CIP) (pp. 26–55). In a nutshell, the CIP is the problem that arises when epidemiological measures of association are *also* interpreted as measures of causal strength. Broadbent defines this as "a measure of the net difference in outcome explained by an exposure" (p. 50).

The term *explanation* is hard to find in the epidemiological literature, but the concept plays an important role in the context of discussions of confounding. Mervyn Susser used the term "explanatory antecedent variable" for a confounder C (Figure 3.1), a common cause that explains the association between a putative cause (exposure E) and its putative effect (outcome O). In such a situation, a common antecedent is a cause of both E and O, thereby explaining why E and O appear to be causally related even if this is not true. In such a case, the net difference in outcome is better explained as a consequence of variable C rather than of variable E.[1]

Epidemiologists concerned with questions about causation and causal inference seem to use the term *explanation* in a slightly different way. For example, Galea, Riddle, and Kaplan come from the complex systems perspective and suggest that

> [i]t would be one small step to move methodologists' thinking from one concerned with fine-tuning methods in the hunt for causes, to incorporating methods that study interrelations and provide explanations for populations as systems. (Galea, Riddle, and Kaplan 2010)

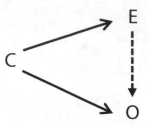

Figure 3.1 Spurious causal inference (dashed arrow) in a situation where an antecedent confounder (C) causes both the putative cause (exposure E) and the putative effect (outcome O).

Although it is not likely that moving methodologists' thinking *anywhere* can be achieved in "one small step," Galea and colleagues have a point when they suggest that providing EEs requires network thinking at the population level by incorporating a multitude of possible exposures and explanatory variables.

Similarly, epidemiologists Mark Parascandola and Douglas Weed think that explanation is a more general, overarching characteristic of epidemiological research:

> Unfortunately, philosophical thinking about causation has been largely driven by the physical sciences, focusing on simple chains of events rather than the complex multi-level relations that make up biology. Thus, this is an area that needs further research. How are explanations at different levels, from the molecular to the social, related? (Parascandola and Weed 2001:911)

Parascandola and Weed are not interested in merely providing a definition of causation for epidemiologists, although they clearly consider this important for everyday epidemiological practice. Instead, they suggest we should find one that "best meets the goals of the discipline of epidemiology."[2]

Briefly outlined in the next two sections are the *textbook* goals of epidemiology, *to identify causes of* illness (Section 3.1.1), and its de facto goal, that is, *to provide useful etiological explanations* (Section 3.1.2). The notions of *macro-* and *micro-etiological* levels of explanation and a sequence of definitions for what is considered to be plain, good, and useful EEs are introduced.[3] Broadbent proposes two characteristics that causal inferences should have in order to serve the needs of epidemiology, stability, and prediction. These are also characteristics of useful EEs. In Section 3.2, a third characteristic is added to the list, *successful intervention*.

3.1.1 Textbook goals of epidemiology

What exactly are the stated goals of epidemiology? Some textbooks state that the goal of epidemiology is *to identify the causes of disease.*[4] In order to do this, epidemiological research needs to provide evidence in support of the conclusion that an observed association between a certain exposure (say, usage of a mobile phone) and a defined health outcome (brain cancer) is, in fact, causal?

Epidemiologist Dimitrios Trichopoulos (1938–2014) expressed his belief that epidemiological results can indeed speak to the issue of causation when he wrote that

> Epidemiology should be evaluated in comparison to other disciplines that serve the same objective, that is, to identify the causes of human disease and facilitate their prevention. Among these disciplines, only epidemiology can document causation without concern about dose-extrapolation or species vabiability [sic] and with built-in accounting for potential modifiers. (Trichopoulos 1995)

Epidemiologist Miguel Hernán, a champion of the potential outcomes approach[5] (POA), agrees: "Population causal effects can sometimes be computed – or, more rigorously, consistently estimated" (Hernán 2004:266). The POA is an approach to causal inference that was cultivated by scholars with backgrounds in statistics[6] and engineering.[7] Its main thrust is based on counterfactual reasoning and goes somewhat like this. A cause makes a difference to its effect. The only way to establish this would be to have a comparison between two scenarios, one in which we observe the occurrence of the effect in the presence of the putative cause versus its absence. Since the *same* event cannot occur twice, we need to resort to *similar* events, and currently the best way to design such similar events (with and without the cause present) devoid of all extraneous influence is *randomization*. The POA is based on the assumption that "the randomized experiment [is] the only scientifically proven method of testing causal relations from data, and to this day, the one and only causal concept permitted in mainstream statistics" (Pearl 2000:340). Even more explicit is Hernán's statement that "in ideal randomized experiments, association *is* causation" (Hernán 2004:267; emphasis mine). The question is, however, how can we identify a cause when we see one?

Epidemiologists have already achieved their textbook goal, to identify causes of illness. However, this is not because of any epistemological technique to extract causal information from observational data. Instead, this is due to their contribution to a larger-scale research process that involves more than one study, multiple kinds of study designs, bench science, sociological research, and so forth. All that epidemiologists can do is look at the beginning and end of the *etiological* process, while their ability to look into what has been called the *black box*, that is, the *pathomechanism*, is limited.[8] This point is revisited in Section 3.2 in a discussion of data manipulation in the service of EEs.

Epidemiologists create explanatory models of disease occurrence in populations that are built on data from epidemiological studies viewed as quasi-real-life scenarios of natural illness occurrence in populations (observational, noninterventional studies). These models, in turn, supplement laboratory data in providing the justification for randomized interventional trials, which are simulations (seeking efficacy) of real-life interventions (yielding effectiveness). In medicine, such interventional studies are considered the "proof of the pudding." However, they are often not perceived as part of the initial discovery process but as playing a more confirmatory role[9] in the overarching scientific process that justifies the approval of drugs by regulatory authorities and the implementation of health policies.

Adding a quantitative twist, it has been suggested that epidemiology's goal is to move beyond identification of causation toward providing a "quantification of the causal relation between exposure and disease" (Savitz 2003:9). For example, Hernán suggests that "the causal risk difference, risk ratio, and odds ratio (and other causal parameters) can also be used to quantify the strength of the causal effect when it exists" (Hernán 2004:267). This statement is problematic in general. In order to quantify something, it has to be measurable, at least in principle. Measurement is the comparison of an observed entity to a reference value. We count our blessings, compare the result to zero, and reflect on what the difference might mean. We measure our body weight and height, calculate our body mass index, compare the result to standard values, and wonder how this could have happened. This may not be possible in the context of illness causation, and perhaps not for any causal context in general. For a cause to be quantifiable, there would need to be a *more or less* or something like a *weak or strong*. This, however, is not really what the concept of cause is all about; something is usually taken to be a cause or it is not, which makes it a categorical concept. In statistical terms, the scale for causation is *nominal* (as in dead or alive), not ordinal (as in stages of breast cancer), or discrete (as in number of joints with arthritis), or even continuous (as in cholesterol level). We do not say that "smoking is a strong cause of lung cancer." We do not compare causes quantitatively, as in "airplane crashes are a weaker cause of death than car accidents." What we talk about is the strength of an association, which in epidemiology increases with an increasing difference between the two scenarios mentioned earlier, between the percentage of individuals with a certain risk factor who develop a particular illness and the percentage of individuals without that same risk factor who develop it. This so-called *risk ratio* (when one is divided by the other) or *risk difference* (if one is subtracted from the other) may be a quantifiable entity, but the causal relationship between risk factor and illness is not.

3.1.2 De facto goal: Useful etiological explanations

Although epidemiologists say that they are searching for causes of illness, they have yet to offer a unified definition of what they mean by *causation* and what a causation detector might look like. Some hope to find causes while admitting that this might be impossible. Broadbent states that uncertainties among epidemiologists about what causation is and what criteria they need to identify causes are irrelevant with regard to their work, because what epidemiologists actually do is generate evidence that helps provide *useful EEs* of illness occurrence.

As mentioned earlier, the arguably most helpful definition of *etiology* is MacMahon and Pugh's, which covers *causal events* that occur before any bodily response and *mechanisms* that lead from the initial bodily response to the first manifestations of illness (MacMahon and Pugh 1970:26). Illness causation is the process that leads from causal events to the biological pathogenetic mechanism. The disease process then develops from pathogenesis to clinical disease. Providing an *EE* is to explain illness occurrence by offering a detailed description of the overarching two-phase etiological process. Giving an EE is more than describing the co-occurrence of an exposure (e.g., asbestos) and outcome (e.g., mesothelioma), which are just the beginning and end of the etiological process. Nobody would consider that offering two photos of the same person, say, as a baby and as a grandmother, is a good way to explain this person's life course. The two snapshots just do not provide any insight of *how* the individual got from there to here. Similarly, one would not consider the observed association between an increase in the stork population around the city of Berlin and the concurrent increase in deliveries outside city hospitals a valid explanation of the process of human reproduction (Hofer, Przyrembel, and Verleger 2004). Ecological data of this sort remain silent about the process between its beginning and end.

Nevertheless, in order to explain the etiology of illness, epidemiological information is needed to establish a potential link between candidate causes (exposures) and illness (outcome), while biological information is needed to explain *how* humans get from there to here. Data about the entire process have to be collected that provide information about both the etiological *macrolevel* (observed risk factors–outcome associations in populations) and the etiological *microlevel* (pathomechanistic observations in the wet lab).[10] This requires collaboration, or at least some knowledge integration, between macrolevel epidemiologists and microlevel scientists. While the former help explain the *why* of illness occurrence by pinpointing candidate causes, the latter help explain the *how* of illness occurrence by pinpointing the pathogenetic mechanism.[11] Only both explanations together, but neither one alone, can provide a sufficient account of the etiological process of illness occurrence.

EE integrates causal, causal-mechanical, and mechanistic explanations as recently reviewed by D. Benjamin Barros:

> [T]he recent literature thus includes three types of accounts of explanation that incorporate causal concepts. Causal explanation generally seeks to explain a phenomenon by providing information about its causal history. [...] Causal-mechanical explanation focuses on explaining the physical connections between causes and effects. Mechanistic explanation adds an additional explanatory layer by seeking to characterize the mechanism that caused the phenomenon. (Barros 2013:456–7)

Barros' explanatory trinity is based on work by Lewis and van Fraassen (causal), Salmon (causal-mechanical), and Bechtel/Abrahamsen, Glennan, Machamer/ Darden/Craver, and Woodward (mechanistic explanations). In the health sciences, *causal* explanations are provided by interpretations of observational epidemiological study results, where risk factors are considered candidate causes (macro-etiology). *Mechanistic* explanations come from empirical laboratory experiments that specify the pathogenetic component of the etiological process (micro-etiology). *Causal-mechanical* explanations integrate information from both kinds of explanation.[12]

Some time ago, my suggestion was that causal inference in public health needs (1) evidence of exposure primacy in humans, (2) evidence of an association between risk factor and illness,[13] (3) experimental biomechanistic evidence, and (4) evidence of public health intervention effectiveness (Dammann and Leviton 2007). In what follows, how these requirements might also fit EEs is outlined. Taking the etiological explanatory stance releases epidemiologists from their perceived responsibility to provide causal certainty, but it also requires them to accept my definition of EEs (at least as a point of departure), and to help define what it means for an EE to be *good* or, even better, *useful*.

In 1957, Abraham Lilienfeld wrote that, in epidemiology and public health,

> a factor may be defined as a cause of a disease, if the incidence of the disease is diminished when exposure to this factor is likewise diminished. (Lilienfeld 1957)

Although Lilienfeld does not explicitly talk about intervention, his definition hints at the practical goal of public health to reduce disease incidence. The upshot of Lilienfeld's position is the assumption that one can reduce disease incidence by reducing exposure to causal risk factors. Standing in the epidemiological tradition that gave rise to this view, the following proposed definitions of what constitutes EEs, in their good and useful forms, are offered:

A proposed definition of *etiological explanation* (EE) is

> *EE:* A plausible description of a set of causes and pathogenetic mechanisms in whose presence illness occurs consistently more frequently than in their absence.

As an example, let's take maternal infection in pregnancy, inflammatory responses in the placenta and the fetal brain, and long-term adverse neurodevelopmental outcomes.[14] In the 1990s, the main explanation of what causes brain damage in many preterm infants was hypoxia-ischemia, that is, lack of oxygen and blood flow to the brain. The major problem was the absence of measurements of oxygen in and blood flow to the brain of preterm infants that may have supported this explanation. In 1997, the author published with Alan Leviton the hypothesis that infection of the mother during pregnancy might lead to neonatal brain damage (macro-etiological observation) via inflammatory responses in placenta and fetal brain (micro-etiological observation). The explanation was *plausible* because maternal infection can lead to inflammation in the placenta and the fetal brain, which in turn can lead to brain damage, via a cascade of inflammatory proteins called *cytokines* that are produced in abundance by body cells in response to infection, are capable of interfering with brain development, and can lead to frank brain tissue damage. The intrauterine infection and brain damage link is further supported by the fact that both are strongly associated with preterm delivery, explaining the clustering of this high-risk constellation in this population. Finally, both inflammation and brain damage occur much more frequently in the presence of maternal intrauterine infection than in its absence.

This EE needs to be supplemented with additional characteristics if it is to be granted the status of *good* EE. In epidemiology and medicine, the goal is to do something about illness occurrence in order to reduce the illness-associated burden to individuals and populations, respectively. Thus, an EE should be plausibly fit for this purpose, and this is proposed as a preliminary definition of a *good etiological explanation* (GEE):

GEE: Any EE that includes modifiable conditions, whose modification is plausibly likely to be associated with a consistent reduction in illness occurrence.

GEEs are perfectly actionable, and that is indeed what is being done when a proposed intervention is tried for the first time in clinical or community-based populations. Once a candidate intervention has been successfully tested and the results indicate that it yields a health benefit, the associated GEE can be promoted from *good* to *useful etiological explanation* (UEE), and can be defined as

UEE: Any EE or GEE whose actual implementation is associated with a consistent reduction of illness occurrence in populations.

Although none of these proposed definitions refers explicitly to causation or mechanisms, both are implicitly involved in the concept of *set of conditions*.

The earlier proposed definitions hinge on the interpretation of terms such as *likelihood, plausibility,* and *consistency.* In the health sciences, such interpretations are provided by the community of researchers who work on related aspects of the etiological story to be told. In the biomedical sciences, this view features prominently in the work of Ludwik Fleck (1896–1961), who conceptualized scientific knowledge generation as "the result of social activity, because the given body of knowledge goes beyond the individual's limitations."[15] It also resonates with the concept of explanatory coherentism, which is the topic of the final chapter of this book.

In light of this proposal, it is time to amend my earlier suggestion that causal inference in public health needs requirements 1–4 presented earlier. The phrase "causal inference in public health needs" should be replaced with something like "useful etiological explanation integrates." It remains to be fully explored whether each single kind of evidence is necessary and only all four of them together are sufficient to constitute a UEE.[16]

Once again, my proposal is that, instead of dreaming up definitions of illness causation and inventing tools for causal inference, epidemiologists should zoom in on helping to find UEEs. I consider this a direct response to Broadbent's suggestion to transition from causation and causal inference in epidemiology to causal explanation. By accepting his

> simple criterion for the causal interpretation of a measure of strength of association: A measure of causal strength is a measure of the net difference in outcome explained by an exposure. (Broadbent 2013:50)

we can return to my earlier proposed definition of UEE and substitute "reduction of" with "net difference in," so that a UEE can now be defined as

UEE: Any EE or GEE whose implementation is associated with a robust net difference in illness occurrence in populations that is explained by the exposure.[17]

Explanation features prominently in Illari and Russo's book, *Causality: Philosophical Theory Meets Scientific Process*, as one of five kinds of problems that "link philosophical theory and scientific practice" (Illari and Russo 2014:5), the other four being inference, prediction, control, and reasoning. Illari and Russo apparently see the term *causal explanation* as including all three explanatory categories in Barros' classification when they state that

> [W]e often want to know not just what happened or will happen, but how it happened, and why. This is causal explanation. (Illari and Russo 2014:262)

They refer to correlations between exposures and outcomes observed in big datasets when they refer to the *what happened* ("exposure to radiation is statistically associated with the occurrence of cancer"). The explanation *how happened what happened* could be either causal-mechanical ("the tumor grew because the exposure to radiation led to DNA double-strand breakage and subsequent proliferation of cancerous cells") or mechanistic ("because of DNA double-strand breakage and subsequent proliferation of cancerous cells"). The explanation *why happened what happened* could be causal ("the tumor grew because of the exposure to radiation") but also causal-mechanical or mechanistic as exemplified earlier. Thus, if Russo and Illari think that asking the *how* and *why* questions is asking for a causal explanation, they implicitly include all three of Barros' kinds of explanation.

In contrast, I think that EEs are helpful precisely *because* they distinguish between causal (macro-etiological) and biomechanistic (micro-etiological) explanations, which play separate roles in public health and medicine, respectively.[18] In public health, the goal of primary prevention and health promotion is reached when a reduction of causes featuring in the causal history of the disease (e.g., less smoking) leads to less (lung) disease occurrence in a population, and this can be achieved without any reference to mechanisms; (macro) EE is all that is needed (Broadbent 2013:77). In secondary prevention and clinical care, however, the pathogenetic mechanism is the target of intervention. Here, causal-mechanical and mechanistic (micro-etiological) explanations of *how* the disease came about (rather than what items in its history gave rise to the circumstances for, and activation of, the mechanism referred to by the word "how") are helpful when it comes to the targeted design of appropriate pharmacological substances that can modify or even interrupt biological processes that characterize specific pathogenetic mechanisms.

Prevention and other kinds of health intervention are things we do to reduce the individual and societal burden associated with illness. This, in turn, motivates us to suggest adding *explanation by intervention* to Broadbent's shortlist of explanatory foci, explanation by stability, and prediction. Therefore, the role of interventions in EEs is now discussed. Described in the next section are three characteristics of the randomized controlled trial (RCT), the interventional study design that is considered the gold standard for causal inference in epidemiology, mainly due to the bias-reducing effects of randomization and blinding. Beyond these two, it is argued that the intervention itself provides added epistemic benefit. Further, it is proposed that even *quasi-interventions* like data analytic manipulations might carry that added benefit. Objections are discussed, and responses are offered.

3.2 EXPLANATION BY INTERVENTION

3.2.1 The gold standard

One of Broadbent's main proposals is to consider steering away from the traditional focus on causal *inference* in epidemiological research toward causal *explanation*. He claims that "good causal inference in epidemiology must deliver a piece of causal knowledge that can be used to improve population health" (Broadbent 2013:56). In particular, he suggests looking for stability and good prediction (SGP) as characteristics of epidemiological results that are capable of contributing to causal explanations.

Broadbent comes from the perspective of Lipton's *inference to the best explanation* (Lipton 1991). He asks for contrastive explanations that tell us "Why this, but not that?" instead of simply "Why this?" Relative risk estimates (outcome risk among exposed individuals divided by outcome risk among the unexposed) require evaluation for SGP before being used for the purpose of causal explanation, because there is nothing in these numbers that allows for causal interpretation. Because EEs consider pathomechanistic evidence, they will be more detailed, finer grained, and more useful in helping us understand how one particular risk factor, but not *that other one*, explains the occurrence of a certain disease. EEs are helpful in supporting the design of new interventions by virtue of explaining why some outcomes are to be expected, while others are not.

As mentioned previously, the gold standard for causal inference in the health sciences is the RCT.[19] In an RCT, two groups of study participants are (1) randomized into two or more treatment groups and (2) exposed to (treated with) either an interventional drug or a placebo (sometimes a different drug). Two crucial characteristics of RCTs are *randomization* and *blinding*. *Randomization* is crucial because it is instrumental in curbing external influence on the causal effect under investigation, thereby sprinkling causal "pixie dust" over an observed association, rendering it causal for all intents and purposes. Here is one example for how the argument is put forward in one of the major epidemiological textbooks:

> Each unit is assigned treatment using a random assignment mechanism such as a coin toss. Such a mechanism is unrelated to the extraneous factors that affect the outcome, so any association between the treatment allocation it produces and those extraneous factors will be random. The variation in the outcome across treatment groups that is not due to treatment effects can thus be ascribed to these random associations and hence can be justifiably called chance variation. (Rothman, Greenland, and Lash 2008b:88)

The idea is that randomization renders the exposure independent of all possible endogenous and exogenous confounding influences. Confounders are characteristics of study participants that are associated with both the exposure and the outcome of interest, for example, a common cause. Any confounder can bias the dataset toward or away from "the null," the numerical measure of "no effect." Randomization is thought of as ascertaining that all confounders are distributed equally among those who receive the intervention and those who do not. Philosopher John Worrall has argued that randomization cannot guarantee the absence of residual confounding

(Worrall 2007) because "the unverifiable assumption of no unmeasured confounding of the exposure effect is necessary for causal inference from observational data" (Hernán and Robins 2006b). And despite all randomization, even RCTs yield only measures of association based on observations. Because "there is no logic that gets you from probabilities or associations alone to causal conclusions" (Kincaid 2011) in observational studies or in RCTs, the latter provide no epistemological impact beyond that provided by the former. Consequently, to consider causal inference based solely on the notion of randomization better than causal inference based on "observational" studies seems to be unjustified.

Randomized studies are *blinded* so that study participants, investigators, and analysts are unaware of the interventional allocation. This reduces bias that is potentially introduced by choices individuals make, especially by choices that could break the randomization scheme and choices that would lead to a violation of the requirement that the outcome should be assessed without knowledge of the outcome. All involved have to be blinded with regard to the exposure, especially those who have a vested interest in the success of the intervention: patients who want to get better, their doctors who want to help, and statisticians and pharmaco-epidemiologists who hope to publish exciting data. If we left interventional allocation to these stakeholders, and one or some of them let their motivation get into the way, the result would be "bias by self-interest." A related bias is "confounding by indication," where the causal effect ascribed to the intervention should better be ascribed to the reasons for the intervention.

Outlined in the next section are some reasons beyond randomization and blinding for why supplementing Broadbent's SGP requirement with data from interventional studies might improve EE. The concept of "quasi-intervention" is presented, and how it can help EEs via data manipulation is discussed.

3.2.2 Intervention

The main reason to propose the concept of *explanation by intervention* is that the successful *prevention* of illness is the ultimate accomplishment in public health. Primary prevention is defined as a reduction of disease incidence (new cases per time unit) and, thereby, disease prevalence (percentage) at the population level. This concept of prevention in public health includes the notion of *intervention*. Therefore, much EE in the population health sciences resonates with Woodward's manipulability theory (Woodward 2003, 2009). In a nutshell, this theory holds that under idealized experimental conditions, X causes Y if there is a possible manipulation of some value of X that leads to a change in Y. This notion is important for EEs, because this is how experimental (micro-etiological) benchwork and RCTs (which are micro- and/or macro-etiological interventions) work: we manipulate X and see if that intervention is associated with a change in Y.

Woodward's rationale for taking this perspective is based on his assumption that "the distinctive practical payoff of causal knowledge has to do with its usefulness for manipulation and control" (Woodward 2003:32). The similarity of the RCT design to that of wet bench experimentation is, according to Woodward, "relevant to establishing causal claims because those claims consist in … claims about what would happen to effects under appropriate manipulations of their putative causes"

(Woodward 2009:35). This reflects exactly what medical and public health researchers are seeking: knowledge about what would happen to health outcomes if their putative causes were manipulated.[20]

One obvious problem for interventionist evidence as a requirement for etiologic explanation is that both lab experiments and RCTs allow for etiological explanation only in those particular manipulationist scenarios, but not in the nonmanipulated "real world." Another problem is the impossibility to infer directly from laboratory animal to humans. Together, these two limitations are the reasons why you cannot go to the lab, induce cerebral damage in newborn mice by injecting a certain substance S into their brains, and then postulate that S is the cause of brain damage in human newborns. Experiments and RCTs yield the information whether a certain manipulation of X *can* cause a change in Y, but they cannot answer the question of whether X causes Y in the real world.[21]

Noninterventional (a.k.a., "observational"[22]) epidemiological studies yield measures of association between exposures and outcomes. Unfortunately, the well-worn notion that "association is not causation" suggests that it is impossible to infer causation from observed association without further ado. Hill's heuristics and the potential outcomes approach (POA) were previously outlined as candidate "causation makers" in epidemiology.[23] Hill's heuristics help to put an observed association into perspective by probing into plausibility, consistency, coherence, and similar characteristics of the observed association between risk factor and outcome.[24] While Hill's heuristics require a comprehensive qualitative content analysis of information from multiple sources and scientific disciplines, the POA puts all its money on the one idea that observation of a quantitative outcome difference in a randomized, controlled experiment allows for a causal interpretation of the relationship between the experimental intervention and the outcome.[25]

Considerable effort is devoted to the avoidance of chance, bias, and confounding during the design, implementation, and analysis phases of observational epidemiological studies. Still, RCTs are often considered superior to observational studies in terms of *causal yield* and, therefore, a more solid basis for success and progress in medicine and public health.[26] Although causal claims based on RCTs are very common in biomedicine, it is difficult to accept statements such as "given fallible access to knowledge of causal processes in the clinical sciences, some epistemic good is provided by conducting randomized interventional studies rather than observational studies" (La Caze 2013). What epistemic benefit can RCTs provide above that provided by observational studies if *all* knowledge of causal processes is fallible? Is it *less* fallible when it is based on data from RCTs instead on observational research? Which characteristic of RCTs can be considered the truth maker in this context? If it is true that "causal inference is just that – an inference by the interpreter of the data, not a product of the study or something that is found within the evidence generated by the study" (Savitz 2003:20), why should data from RCTs enable the interpreter to draw valid causal inference while data from observational studies fail to do so?

One important argument against this recipe for cause-making is that, after all is said and done, experimental results are also just observations. Why should observation of postinterventional occurrence of health phenomena be epistemologically superior to observation of natural or free-floating occurrence?

First, observation of manipulated occurrence in humans may be considered epistemologically superior to the observation of natural or free-floating occurrence in natural experiments or in observational epidemiological studies, because it comes with the added benefit of providing evidence of *efficacy*, which suggests that the intervention would work (or not) in the real-life setting of medical or public health interventions. RCTs are conducted in humans; they involve the administration of real drugs, and they measure real outcomes. If a drug works in an RCT, it is likely that it will also work in a real-life setting. This added benefit is not provided by randomization or blinding alone, which are characteristics of RCTs that make them less like real-life interventions; the manipulation makes the observed phenomena in RCTs more like real-life medical or public health interventions.

Second, my suggestion to complement Broadbent's SGP requirement with evidence from intervention is motivated by the recognition that even if we already have stable and predictive information from cohort or case-control studies, EE would be *better* if we had additional evidence from intervention. While observation of free-floating occurrence yields data for basic EEs, observation of manipulated occurrence yields data for UEEs that may justify clinical or public health interventions, precisely *because* it is evidence from intervention, the target for most epidemiological knowledge generation (Dammann 2015).

The lack of results from interventional studies can also be quite enlightening. For example, it is entirely conceivable that an epidemiological result is stable and predictive in multiple observational studies (Flanders et al. 2011a, 2011b), but clinical trials fail to result in the expected change in the outcome after intervention on the exposure variable. One prominent example is the initial finding in the Nurses' Health Study that postmenopausal estrogen use is associated with a reduced risk for coronary heart disease over a 4-year follow-up period (Stampfer et al. 1985). Half a decade later, 10-year follow-up data confirmed these results (Stampfer et al. 1991). However, a subsequent randomized trial did not show a benefit (Hulley et al. 1998), and this result was more recently confirmed by meta-analytic approaches (Main et al. 2013). Had the randomized estrogen trial not contradicted observational results, for how long would we have thought about estrogen as a means to prevent cardiovascular disease in postmenopausal women? The observational result was rather stable over time (in that same cohort); however, we are lucky that a comparably large observational cohort study (the Framingham study) existed at that time, had the necessary data available, and did *not* show a protective effect (Wilson, Garrison, and Castelli 1985). This is the kind of situation that warrants a clinical trial (i.e., a situation of uncertainty regarding efficacy called *equipoise*) to resolve the tension that arises due to incongruent results from observational studies of similar quality.

Broadbent's requirement for stability of an observational epidemiological result is that

(a) it is not soon contradicted by good scientific evidence, and (b) given best current scientific knowledge, it would probably not be soon contradicted by good scientific evidence, if good research were done on the topic. (Broadbent 2013:63)

In the context of large-scale, population-based, prospective studies, one problem with part (a) of this requirement is that it is highly unlikely that *any* result from *any* comparable study will be available soon, just because these studies are so expensive, time consuming, and difficult to implement. A problem with part (b) is that in many cases we simply cannot tell what might happen if good research were done.

If a cohort study does *not* yield an interesting result, only very few hardliners will embark on the long journey of conducting another, similar study without solid preliminary data. If they do, it will take years, if not decades until the results are in. If, on the other hand, a cohort study *does* yield an interesting result, it is likely that, for the sake of saving time and money, investigators move on to the RCT right away. In either case, it is quite unlikely that a comparable observational study will be performed just to confirm or contradict the initial results. *Confirmation* of results of successful observational studies by similarly successful RCTs, however, comes at almost no cost, because interventional design is why observational studies are performed in the first place.[27]

Third, manipulation reduces the inferential margin of error induced by confounding factors. While the observed association between intervention and outcome might still be due to chance, any confounding factor (i.e., a common cause of intervention and outcome) would need to influence the manipulator's agency and independently influence the outcome. It could be argued that candidate confounders would, thus, boil down factors that influence the manipulator's decision:

- At which explanatory level to intervene (macro- or micro-etiological levels by intervening on risk factors or pathogenetic mechanisms, respectively), thereby putting constraints on her inference by limiting the realm of her predictions about consequences to that level.
- At what point in time to intervene and for how long, thereby putting constraints on her inference with regard to the time frame for expected changes in outcome.
- How intensely to intervene (e.g., drug dosage), thereby putting constraints on her inference in terms of dose-response relationships between intervention and outcome.

Investigators can deliberately vary timing, duration, and dosage of the intervention and observe changes in the outcome. If changes in outcome are associated with changes in manipulated exposure, it seems more plausible that we "made" those changes in outcome by changing the treatment regimen.[28] Always, however, the possibility remains that all such changes occur solely by chance.

Finally, it could be that investigators simply prefer to rely on what they observe "with their own eyes" in a system's behavior after they have manipulated it "with their own hands" rather than rely on what they passively observe in the system's behavior, because intervention appears to be a quintessential component of the way we learn about causation (Gopnik and Schulz 2007). In everyday situations, we gather causal knowledge about how the world around us works by paying attention to how our actions (or our avoidance thereof) modify the trajectory of events and, thereby, potential outcomes of situations. Perhaps we simply prefer evidence from intervention because we personally rely on such evidence in our daily lives, all the time.

3.2.3 Quasi-intervention

The notion of "quasi-intervention" concerns *analytical data manipulation* in observational (noninterventional) studies. It builds on the notion that an ideal observational study with sufficient statistical power, well-defined groups of participants, collection of high-quality data, inclusion of all known confounders, and exclusion of all known biases should *not* be considered epistemologically inferior to a randomized trial. The results of a perfect observational study should come rather close to those of a randomized trial. For example, if taking a certain drug has a particular effect on clinical improvement in an *ideal* observational study, the results should be similar to those an RCT would provide. Obviously, it is easy to raise the objection that perfect studies do not exist. However, two data-manipulation techniques, *propensity score adjustment* and *Mendelian randomization* can bring observational study very close to the ideal, thereby contributing to the causal inference part of etiological explanations. A third technique, data stratification, is used to explore a phenomenon called *effect modification*, the observation that effect sizes differ in subgroups of the original study population, indicating that the variable that defines the subgroups must play some kind of mechanistic role in disease etiology.

In some cases, it is impossible for ethical, financial, or timing reasons to conduct a RCT. For this scenario, epidemiologists and statisticians have developed a data analysis tool called *propensity score*. Once the data are in, information on all confounders is used to calculate a score that allows the investigator to adjust for all confounders by matching or adjusting in multivariable regression models. The idea is to make exposed and unexposed groups as similar as possible, and indeed as similar as the groups in a randomized trial. Any potential bias due to stakeholder motivation or confounding by indication can be minimized in this way. In some settings, such propensity score-adjusted observational studies are not only the best we can do, but *the only thing* we can do to emulate the design features of a randomized trial. It is impossible to conduct both kinds of study in the same population. However, even if it were possible, there is no external gold standard each study could be compared to. Thus, any claim that RCTs are genuinely better than propensity score-adjusted observational studies remains unsupported. Thus, retroactive propensity score calculation and adjustment is considered a plausible simulation of randomization in an RCT.

Mendelian randomization is a more recently developed technique in which investigators identify a genetic variant that is strongly biologically associated with the exposure under investigation. Study participants are then divided into groups defined by the presence or absence of that same genetic variant. Since genetic traits are inherited in a random fashion, the groups are now effectively randomized; confounders are distributed equally between groups, and results turn out to be very close to those from a randomized trial (Yarmolinsky et al. 2018).

Effect modification is a phenomenon that is neither a bias to be avoided, nor a kind of confounding to be adjusted for; it is a biological characteristic that leads to different effect sizes in strata of the study population defined by the effect modifier.[29] Stratified data analysis is one way to explore effect modification. For example, the association between obesity and stillbirth was only modestly elevated among Black women (relative risk 1.1), slightly stronger in White women (1.3), and prominently stronger among Asian women (4.6) (Penn et al. 2014). Although the biological inferences to be drawn upon post hoc effect modification analyses may be quite limited (Thompson 1991), there is very little support for the contention that, if all data are carefully collected prospectively, there is any epistemological difference between the results of effect modification analysis after *a priori* versus *a posteriori* stratification. In my view, it simply does not matter whether we organize exposed and unexposed in strata defined by the effect modifier variable before or after data collection is completed.

Now consider the question whether evidence from intervention by data manipulation can be considered epistemologically equivalent to evidence from real-life intervention. Note that we are not asking the question whether conclusions based on observational studies are similar to those based on randomized studies,[30] but whether conclusions based on observational studies are similar to conclusions based on interventional ones, the contrast being the intervention (manipulation), not the randomization. If yes, does this qualify only as evidence of the confirmatory kind, or does it also qualify as evidence of the kind that informs etiological explanations from observational data by alluding to micro-etiological mechanisms?

To answer the first question, *there is no real-life equivalent to data manipulation.* Real-life intervention means to proactively change the life course of human individuals and collect data on outcomes prospectively; data manipulation is just playing retrospectively with numbers that are already collected, albeit in a very meaningful way. In fact, the data are not manipulated in the sense of being changed but just organized in strata defined by, for example, potential effect modifiers or confounders. My point is that an observed association between E and O can be modified and perhaps further clarified by comparing scenarios such as E → O with confounder adjustment versus without, or E → O in the entire study sample versus in subgroups. In this way, manipulation of observational data can contribute to the elucidation of etiological mechanisms[31] and, thereby, contribute to the mechanistic component of etiological explanation from observation.[32]

The opportunity to compare randomized and nonrandomized studies directly is obviously limited to exposure variables that have in fact been evaluated in both kinds of study. This will exclude risk factors that are ethically impossible to study in an RCT and also potentially preventive or therapeutic interventions that cannot be studied in cross-sectional, cohort, or case-control studies, for whatever reason.

3.2.4 Objections

Three major objections to my explanation-by-intervention suggestion are (1) a *circularity* objection, (2) a *temporality* objection, and (3) an *incompatibility* objection.

First, if the goal is to assign explanatory value to an observed effect measure derived from a successful interventional study, it seems *circular* to require such a result in order to establish the prediction that an intervention should be successful.[33] The circularity objection holds that interventional results cannot inform causal explanations based on results from observational studies because observational studies yield a good causal explanation only if the prediction they support (that a randomized trial should be successful) is confirmed by a successful intervention trial. Agreement to this objection can be made to the extent that interventional results cannot inform a causal explanation from observations that is used to justify that same interventional trial. However, it can be used to inform a causal explanation that serves as the justification for any *subsequent* interventional study.[34] This is part of the process of mounting the observational and interventional evidence in support of the *overarching causal explanation and related prediction* that "exposure E causes outcome O and therefore intervention on E will successfully prevent or at least ameliorate O."

Second, the *temporality* objection holds that an intervention can only confirm, not explain, because information from interventional studies becomes available only if causal inference from observational studies appears already robust enough to the scientific community so that an interventional trial seems justified. The usual etiological research workflow has observational studies most often preceding interventional studies. Results from the latter become available only years, sometimes decades after the first observational results are available. Therefore, interventional data cannot inform an etiological explanation based on observational data simply because they become available only *after* the causal conclusion they are supposed to inform has already been drawn.

Third, the *incompatibility* objection to the proposal to add evidence from intervention to etiological explanations is that doing so is impossible because interventional studies (apples) are not observational studies (oranges) and, therefore, cannot inform causal claims based on observational data. The objection essentially maintains that interventional studies are not only epistemologically superior to observational studies but also epistemologically *different*. The randomized trial is methodologically similar to a controlled laboratory experiment in simple systems, where the exposure in randomly selected individuals is allocated by the investigators and does not occur freely in a population without any external manipulation (as in observational studies). Therefore, interventional results cannot really inform causal explanations from observation but can only either confirm or contradict them.

Although not all will agree that results from interventional studies can enhance causal explanation based on observational studies, they can (and do) enhance the entire overarching research program, which is to provide useful etiological explanations. If "the determination that an association is causal indicates the possibility for intervention" (Glass et al. 2013), that indication would be even more justified if based on etiological explanations that include evidence from interventions. Either one alone can provide an etiological explanation, but observational and interventional epidemiology together will provide a stronger one. If interventional data cannot contribute to the first draft of a particular etiological explanation, they can certainly contribute to its revision and refinement.

Observational epidemiology, wet bench science, and interventional studies can form a stepwise process of generating a useful etiological explanation. The logic of the research program would go like this:

E explains a net difference in O because (i) observational epidemiologic studies suggest that E and O are potentially causally associated. Therefore, bench experiments are

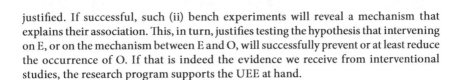

justified. If successful, such (ii) bench experiments will reveal a mechanism that explains their association. This, in turn, justifies testing the hypothesis that intervening on E, or on the mechanism between E and O, will successfully prevent or at least reduce the occurrence of O. If that is indeed the evidence we receive from interventional studies, the research program supports the UEE at hand.

This procedure may be viewed as sidestepping the apples and oranges point, the point that interventional studies are inherently different from observational studies and therefore cannot inform causal explanations from observational studies, only confirm them. However, part of the motivation for this move is my perception that we are always likely to miss something if we do not look at all the "evidential variety" (Claveau 2012) summarized as the "explanatory story" (Haack 2004), characterized by "robustness, the state in which a hypothesis is supported by evidence from multiple techniques with independent background assumptions" (Stegenga 2009:651).

Etiological explanation based on results from laboratory, epidemiology, and interventional trials is arguably more robust than evidence based on results from the lab and from observational epidemiology alone. The discussion offered in this section supports my suggestion that the statement

E explains a net difference in O because (i) we have an observed association between the two, and (ii) we have a mechanism that explains how they are related.[35]

is considerably weaker than this one:

E explains a net difference in O because (i) we have an observed association between the two, and (ii) we have a mechanism that explains how they are related, and intervention on E changes the risk of O.

In sum, I think that results from interventional studies both inform and confirm etiological explanations in the context of comprehensive multidisciplinary research programs whose goal is to come up with new health interventions that work. Such projects are usually long term, multidisciplinary, and require theory *plus* epidemiological observation *plus* lab experiment *plus* clinical trial *plus* postmarketing effectiveness studies. Such projects never zoom in on the epidemiology-centered silver-bullet approaches but like a mosaic of evidence (see Chapter 4), because "the structure of evidence is not linear, like a mathematical proof, but ramifies like a crossword puzzle" (Haack 2004).

4 ETIOLOGICAL PLURALISM

4.1 INTRODUCTION

In the previous chapter, the idea that etiological explanations might be more helpful than causal inference was advocated, in part because etiological explanations are causal-mechanical explanations. But if mechanisms play such an important role, what are these mechanisms? How are they related to their causes? Are all these mechanisms similar or even the same? How about the notion that, particularly in biomedicine, not all causes and mechanisms can be the same, because we often talk about social, environmental, genetic, and psychological causes and mechanisms. Is it possible that all of these are the same?

In Section 4.2, the mosaicist view offered by Phyllis Illari and Federica Russo (2014) is considered. Their book provides an excellent introduction to accounts of causality and arrives at the conclusion that "the idea of developing One True Causal Theory is not promising" (p. 247). Instead, the authors propose embracing a "cheerful conceptual pluralism" that employs "*all the developed accounts and theories in the literature*" (p. 256; italics in original) They think that taking a stab at causation in the sciences requires a pluralist perspective, simply because the sheer variety of causal concepts and methods in the sciences just cannot fit under a monist umbrella. Here their suggestion is taken and applied to etiological explanations (Section 4.3), and etiological pluralism is proposed as pluralism about the real-world phenomenon of the illness causation process, not about a variety of concepts about it (Section 4.4). Examples of how etiological pluralism may be conceptualized are offered from the author's area of interest (perinatal neuroinflammation) (Section 4.5).

4.2 MOSAICIST ARGUMENT

In *Causality: Philosophical Theory Meets Scientific Practice*, Illari and Russo propose that, perhaps, looking at many different characterizations of causality, arranged like a mosaic[1] might provide more insight than looking at each one individually. They present five scientific problems they consider important motivations to bring together philosophical theory and scientific practice: Inference (Does X cause Y?), prediction (What will happen?), explanation (How does X cause Y?), control (How to control causal systems?), and reasoning about causality. They discuss a whole host of specific notions of causality, for example, necessary/sufficient, probabilism, counterfactuals, manipulation, processes, mechanisms, information, dispositions, regularity, variation, action, inference, and others. With regard to epidemiology and medicine, they mention the problem of criteria for illness causation, the problem of causes versus conditions of illness, and the problem of illness in individuals versus populations.

Illari and Russo illustrate how closely related the philosophical and epidemiological ways of thinking about causality can be. They show that Ken Rothman's model (called the Mackie–Rothman model in Section 2.4.1) of sufficient constellations of insufficient component causes[2] is in fact an epidemiological adaptation of Mackie's INUS conditions: Insufficient nonredundant parts of unnecessary but sufficient causes (Mackie 1965, 1974). The Rothman model conceives of sufficient causes of illness (C_{si}) as constellations of component causes (c_{ci}), for example, $C_{s1} \equiv [c_{c1}, c_{c2}, c_{c3}, c_{c4}]$, $C_{s2} \equiv [c_{c1}, c_{c4}, c_{c5}, c_{c6}]$, $C_{s3} \equiv [c_{c1}, c_{c6}, c_{c7}, c_{c8}]$. Let us assume that C_{s1}, C_{s2}, and C_{s3} account for equally sized proportions of all causes of the disease of interest; each one causes one-third (33.3%) of all cases. Note that *none* of the three sufficient causes (or better, causal constellations) is *necessary* for the disease to occur. Also note that none of the component causes alone is sufficient, and only c_{c1} is necessary because none of the sufficient causal constellations is complete without c_{c1}. All other component causes are insufficient *and* unnecessary. The philosophical parallel here is that each one of the component causes c_{c1-7} qualifies as a Mackiean INUS condition.

In another example, Illari and Russo turn to semantic differences between the philosophical and scientific terminology. They write about levels of causation and the not so obvious difference between the type/token distinction in philosophy and the person/population distinction in medicine and epidemiology. While the former distinguishes between events that recur with some regularity (e.g., the phenomenon of earthquakes) and a single instant (one particular earthquake), the latter distinguishes between population-level occurrence (e.g., the annual incidence of myocardial infarcts in Germany in 1995) and person-level occurrences (my Godfather's myocardial infarct there that same year). Illari and Russo suggest bridging the levels and the terminology (p. 41) by replacing both dyads with the terms "generic" and "single case."

To promote cross-disciplinary communication, Illari and Russo introduce and compare two approaches to causality in philosophy and the sciences. First, they describe how scientists use models to tackle causation. They suggest that it "is not so much whether models allow us to establish the *truth* of a causal claim, but rather whether they are of any *use* for a given problem" (p. 229; italics in original). Second, they write about the identification by philosophers of so-called truthmakers, that is, what it is in the world that makes causal claims true. In their comparison of the truthmaking and modeling approaches, Illari and Russo suggest that

> [w]e'll know whether [a] proposition is in fact true or not by checking the world out there. [...] But prior to empirical investigation, why should we suppose that the reality we are interested in has a rigid constraint on what the causal relation and its relata must be? Indeed, the reasons for pluralism about causality we examine [...] suggest that we have evidence that it cannot be. Allying this with the arguments in the truthmakers literature, we suggest the release of the "One Truth" straightjacket on the truthmakers approach. The resulting picture changes enormously! (p. 233)

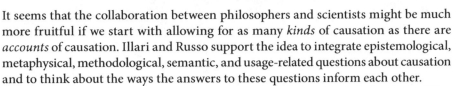

It seems that the collaboration between philosophers and scientists might be much more fruitful if we start with allowing for as many *kinds* of causation as there are *accounts* of causation. Illari and Russo support the idea to integrate epistemological, metaphysical, methodological, semantic, and usage-related questions about causation and to think about the ways the answers to these questions inform each other.

They proceed in two steps. First, they defend their version of pluralism. They offer what they call a "cheerful conceptual pluralism," which draws upon "*all the developed accounts and theories in the literature*" (p. 256; italics in original). They call their form of pluralism *the pluralist mosaic*, borrowing the term from Carl Craver (2007),[3] who used it to suggest that "the mosaic unity of neuroscience is achieved both through interfield integration at a given level and through integration across levels in a hierarchy of mechanisms" (Craver 2007:228). While Craver's *mosaic unity* (of neuroscience) captures a scenario in which different fields of neuroscience contribute different kinds of evidence with different forms of constraints toward "integrated piecemeal as research progresses" (Illari and Russo 2014:231), Illari and Russo envision an even broader mosaicism, one of integration across the sciences and philosophy, across types of causing, concepts of causation, types of inferences, sources of evidence, and across methods for causal inference. They are pragmatists in that they are task oriented: "different concepts help in building causal knowledge, in virtue of their usefulness for specific tasks" (p. 257).

As a second step in supporting their argument, Illari and Russo offer an example of how causal mosaicism can be used in practice. They describe "exposomics" as "the science of exposure"[4] (p. 260) performed by multiple research groups from various fields, rooted in molecular epidemiology using biomarkers of exposure, internal responses, and outcome,[5] and integrating knowledge from all biomedical, basic, and social sciences (p. 264). They demonstrate how to select accounts of causality that might be useful when assembled as a mosaic. Their hope that this approach will help us to "think better about science" (p. 271) is shared.

At this point, the main question is what contribution their pluralist *mosaic* approach to causality will make for scientists and philosophers. It is important to note that the mosaic approach is just that: an *approach* that appreciates all available accounts of causality in an attempt to help clarify (identify and refine) scientific questions and problems (p. 270). It is *not* a novel account of causality that can be compared to currently available accounts. Instead, the proposed model might help scientists and philosophers *to do better work* by helping them to *think better about their work.*

4.3 ETIOLOGICAL PLURALISM

Illari and Russo's emphasis is on what they call a "cheerful conceptual pluralism" of causal modeling. They state that

> the idea of developing One True Causal Theory is not promising. Philosophically minded scientists and scientifically oriented philosophers ought instead to engage in the enterprise of filling in the huge causal mosaic of empirical studies and theoretical investigations … in order to see the whole picture. (p. 247)

Illari and Russo propose a pluralism of pluralisms: of types of causing, of concepts of causation, of types of inferences, of sources of evidence, and of measures for causal inference. They describe each pluralism and write that *all* published accounts and theories (i.e., all pluralisms) can be resources for those who want to think about the sciences (p. 256). They do not really say *why exactly* they think that a pluralism of pluralisms is the way to go but state that

> no single theory of causality currently available can meet the very varied needs of the sciences, and address the problems of causal reasoning, inference, explanation, prediction and control in all the diverse cases that we meet in the sciences. (p. 250)

The advantage of permitting all kinds of pluralisms as pieces for their causal mosaic is that it maximizes the *explanatory potential* of any Illari-Russoian causal mosaic, because there is a large number of possibilities of how elements of all kinds of pluralisms can be combined to form an explanation. Unfortunately, its disadvantage is that such a liberal approach also minimizes the explanatory power for the same reason, because the quality of any explanation needs to be evaluated in comparison to other explanations. The large number of available possible comparisons will keep us busy comparing explanations for a long time.[6]

The notion of causal pluralism in the health sciences might require more than support for the contention *that* the roles causal factors play in the story of illness occurrence are fundamentally different. Addressed in this section is what we mean by *causal pluralism* in the context of etiological explanations. One possibility is to think of causes as being not one, but multiple, fundamentally different *things*. Another possibility is to think of causes as multiple, fundamentally different *ideas*.[7] Causal pluralism in etiological contexts refers to real-life phenomena, not just ideas. The discussion in this chapter makes it clear that in the context of etiological explanations, what we mean by *causal pluralism* is *pluralism of causation*, which includes both a plurality of causes and a plurality of pathomechanisms (Section 4.4). In Section 4.5, one example of pathomechanism is outlined from the *perinatal inflammatory response*, and some of its components are matched to different kinds of antecedents of illness as defined by Susser (Susser 1973). This provides support for the notion that etiological pluralism is *pluralism regarding the real-world phenomenon of how various causes contribute to illness occurrence* via *various pathomechanisms*, not a pluralism of concepts of etiological explanation.

One way of thinking about causal pluralism is to consider different kinds of *causes*. Another is to consider multiple, fundamentally different kinds of *causation*. Apparently, this is what some philosophers mean when they talk about causal pluralism: pluralism not of causes, but of causation; pluralism not of what causes *are*, but of what they *do*. For example, Godfrey-Smith refers to causal pluralism as "the view that causation is not a single kind of relation or connection between things in the world [but] irreducibly plural or diverse" (Godfrey-Smith 2009:326–7). The same holds true for another kind of pluralism that has been added to the mix by Julian Reiss[8]: "*evidential pluralism* [is] the thesis that there are more than one reliable ways to find out about causal relationships"[9] (Reiss 2011:908).

The notion that causal pluralism is about what causes do, not what they are, is supported by the observation that causation is rarely defined using nouns, rather by using verbs that describe the *process of causation*. For example, one perfectly circular definition of causation goes like this: "Causality means that one of the variables actually causes the other" (Waldron 2018:149). Illari and Russo list as examples of causation verbs such as "pulling, pushing, blocking, sticking, breaking, lifting, falling." They also note that all these descriptors have a richer content than "causing," by indicating how the causing is achieved (p. 250). This notion goes back to Anscombe's classic proposal that perhaps "the word 'cause' can be *added* to a language in which are already represented many causal concepts [like] *scrape, push, wet, carry, eat, burn* …" (Anscombe 1993:93; italics in original). This would mean that there are different kinds of processes for which we have different names that we unify linguistically under the term *cause*. Anscombe takes her view to the extreme by imagining a language that has no notions of these different kinds of causal processes; in such language, she holds, "no description of the use of a word […] will be able to present it as meaning *cause*" (ibid.).

As outlined earlier and discussed in more detail in Chapter 7, etiology is the transition from health to illness, characterized by causes that initiate a pathomechanism (causation process), which in turn represents the first stages of the disease itself, which lead to clinically perceivable illness (disease process). This view, called the *etiological stance*,[10] yields etiological explanations, which are explanations that refer to certain causes of illness on one hand, and to their pathomechanisms on the other, as two separate issues. One requires the identification of causes (e.g., maternal infection during pregnancy), and the other requires the identification of pathomechanisms (e.g., a fetal inflammatory response). If causal pluralism is, as Godfrey-Smith and Reiss suggest, a pluralism regarding the "relation or connection between things" and "causal relationships," respectively, causal pluralism in etiological explanations is actually pluralism of illness causation. While the etiological stance separates causes from pathogenesis, it reunites them under the umbrella causation process (see Figure 4.1, which is identical to Figure 7.1). This way we can establish that causal pluralism in the context of etiological explanations is a pluralism of *causation processes*. Still, we need to clarify which part of the causation process is plural: The causal part, the pathogenetic part, or both?

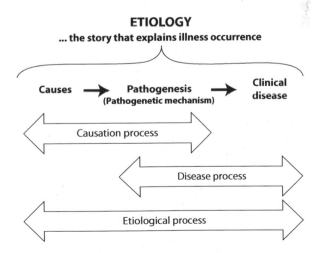

Figure 4.1 The etiological stance. (Reprinted from Dammann O. 2017. *Perspect Biol Med*;60(2):151–65.)

4.4 IN ETIOLOGICAL EXPLANATIONS, CAUSAL PLURALISM IS PLURALISM OF CAUSATION

4.4.1 Pluralism of causes

Let us begin with the causal part. The etiological stance envisions illness occurrence to be the culmination of a sequence of overlapping processes, the causation process and the disease process. This sequence is initiated by *causes* (Figure 4.1).

It is not difficult to distinguish fundamentally different *kinds of causes* of illness. Indeed, fundamental differences between causes of illness are readily apparent and perhaps even trivial. In fact, it seems obvious that car accidents, excessive exposure to sunlight, and inborn genetic variants are very different kinds of things. For example, the first two (accidents, radiation) involve events that happen outside the human body, which is not true for the third (genetics).

The following is an example of how illness occurrence is explained in epidemiology and medicine, provided by scientific staff of the Mayo Clinic in Rochester, Minnesota, who explain cancer occurrence to the public:

> Cancer is caused by changes (mutations) to the DNA within cells. The DNA inside a cell is packaged into a large number of individual genes, each of which contains a set of instructions telling the cell what functions to perform, as well as how to grow and divide. Errors in the instructions can cause the cell to stop its normal function and may allow a cell to become cancerous. [...] Gene mutations can occur for several reasons, for instance:
>
> - Gene mutations you're born with. You may be born with a genetic mutation that you inherited from your parents. This type of mutation accounts for a small percentage of cancers.
> - Gene mutations that occur after birth. Most gene mutations occur after you're born and aren't inherited. A number of forces can cause gene mutations, such as smoking, radiation, viruses, cancer-causing chemicals (carcinogens), obesity, hormones, chronic inflammation and a lack of exercise.
> - Gene mutations occur frequently during normal cell growth. However, cells contain a mechanism that recognizes when a mistake occurs and repairs the mistake. Occasionally, a mistake is missed. This could cause a cell to become cancerous.[11]

Although the Mayo Clinic's explanation starts with "cancer is caused by," it first refers to the *pathomechanism*, which includes gene mutations and abnormal cell growth, as early, subclinical stages of illness. Only then does it refer back to prenatal (inborn, inherited) and postnatal *causes* of gene mutations. Thus, we can distinguish between two fundamentally different kinds of cause, based on *inheritance* – which separates causes that just happen to us without further action on our part from causes that occur after birth. While the former, genetic causes, are related to who we are, the latter are also related to where we live, what we do, and so forth. For example, the American College of Medical Genetics and Genomics has published a guideline for reproductive screening in the Ashkenazi Jewish population (Monaghan et al. 2008) based on the recognition that at least 18 diseases (including cancers of the breast, ovary, and colon) occur more frequently in predominantly Ashkenazi Jewry than in other populations (Ostrer 2001). This risk increase is present from the moment of conception, as opposed to risk increases, which are initiated after birth via causes such as smoking, radiation, viruses, and so forth. Although we may say that the pathomechanism (gene mutation) is the same for inherited and acquired genetic disorders, the causal initiation (fusion of egg and sperm versus later mutation, respectively) is clearly different, as are the diseases themselves. While cystic fibrosis is a disease of the inborn-genetic kind, many forms of cancer are of the acquired-genetic kind, in which the responsible gene mutation occurs in response to exposure such as smoking, radiation, or viruses, which lead to full-blown cancer over longer stretches of time, that is, months, sometimes years, or even decades.[12] Few will find acknowledging such *pluralism of causes* more problematic than acknowledging a pluralism of wildflowers.

4.4.2 Pluralism of causation

A much more interesting way to think about fundamental differences between illness causation processes is to think about fundamental differences between *pathogenetic mechanisms*. This is the process of *how* causes initiate, facilitate, and predispose to illness. These kinds of processes are important for the health sciences, because if elimination of a cause to prevent illness occurrence cannot be achieved, interfering with the disease occurrence *process* might still be an option.[13]

Again, for causes to make a difference with regard to illness occurrence, it is not so much what they *are*, but what they *do*. Mervyn Susser (1921–2014) was one of the few epidemiologists who devoted part of his career to thinking about causality. He begins his 1973 book *Causal Thinking in the Health Sciences* not with a definition of *cause*, but of the term *determinant* as "any factor, whether event, characteristic, or other definable entity, so long as it brings about change for the better or worse in a health condition" (Susser 1973:3). Although this definition does not endorse causal pluralism *expressis verbis*, it suggests that if *any* entity can be conceived of as a determinant of health, there should be different ways in which these antecedents can do the bringing-about-change part, unless they are all doing it in the same way. In fact, Susser distinguishes different *forms of determination*, including *host reactions* (causes that produce the effect), *attributes/predispositions* (causes that predispose to the effect), *preconditions* (a sine qua non cause), and *immanence and heritability* (causes that are programmed into a system that displays the effect). He recognizes that some might not be willing to consider examples for the latter three categories of causes; he lists sex, race, and age as attributes, male sex as a precondition for prostate cancer, and the ability to walk and talk as immanent and heritable. Still, even if we do not feel comfortable calling these characteristics causes, they are definitely candidates for the role of component cause in the Mackie–Rothman model discussed in Section 2.4.1, and perhaps even *necessary* component causes such as piece A in all three pies in Figure 2.2 or the component cause c_{c1} mentioned at the beginning of this chapter. (This would make sense at least for preconditions like male sex for prostate cancer.[14])

4.4.3 Causes versus conditions

Susser's four kinds of cause/determinant can be thought of as playing different *roles* in the process of illness causation. For example, the host reaction kind *produces* the effect, while the precondition kind *provides a necessary background* condition. The distinction between producing causes and background conditions has been, and probably still is, a matter of debate. Mill thought of *the cause* of an event as "the sum total of the conditions positive and negative taken together [...] which being realized, the consequent invariably follows" (Mill 1856:217). Concerns regarding determinist versus probabilist notions in the "invariably follows" part aside, this concept of cause as the sum total of all conditions is reflected in epidemiology in the Mackie–Rothman model.[15]

Broadbent has proposed the term *problem of causal selection* for "the problem of providing an account of the difference between cause and condition" (Broadbent 2008). He holds that a simple counterfactual notion like Lewis' (1973) cannot provide such an account: if C is a cause of effect E, then E does not occur if C does not occur beforehand ($\sim$C > $\sim$E; $\sim$ indicating negation). Broadbent suggests that this counterfactual cannot distinguish between cause and (noncausal) mere condition, because it cannot tell us which one *makes a difference* between fact and counterfactual (and thus is the cause) and which one does not (the mere condition). This reference to difference-making is based on a contrastive account of causation proposed by Peter Lipton (1954–2007); the quote from Lipton that Broadbent provides is: "... a cause marks a difference between the situation where the effect occurs and a contrasting situation where it does not" (Lipton 1992:136). Thus, the difference between fact and counterfactual is defined by the presence or absence of E, not C. In the Lewisean scenario, conversely, the *fact* is the occurrence of C and the *counterfactual* situation is $\sim$C, and what "makes" the difference between these two situations is E, not C. Obviously, this is not the information we are looking for as support for any decision about C as a cause or condition.

In order to see whether C makes (and marks) a difference between fact (E) and counterfact ($\sim$E), we have to take a detour. Broadbent proposes *the Reverse Counterfactual* that holds that if C is a cause of E, then if E had not occurred ($\sim$E), then C would not have occurred ($\sim$C). He states that "the Reverse Counterfactual provides a good analysis of the sense in which causes make a difference to their effects" (Broadbent 2008:360). As an example, he sets up a hypothetical scenario in which he (Broadbent) strikes a match in the presence or absence of oxygen. Although it is true that both not striking the match (cause) and not having oxygen available (condition) would contribute to a situation in which the match does not light, he says that reverse counterfactual analysis can clarify which one is the cause because it makes a difference regarding the match lighting or not. He has us imagine him in his dry and warm kitchen. He strikes a match, and the match lights. The factual situation here is that the match lights, and the corresponding counterfactual situation is one in which the match does not light. Now, Broadbent holds that in the closest counterfactual world, it is more likely that the match was not struck, not that there is no oxygen in the room. On this account, (not) striking the match made the difference, not the absence of oxygen.

Broadbent offers multiple caveats that put his proposal into perspective, including restriction to necessary causes, overdetermination, and the problem of backtracking counterfactuals, among others. For more discussion, see Chapter 7, in which conditions feature prominently. For the time being, this approach might not be of much help in etiological explanations that include the concept of effect modification, in which certain conditions modify causal effects.

In the next section of this chapter, the etiology of neurodevelopmental disorders among preterm newborns is discussed as an example of how Susser's kinds of determinant/determination are aligned with kinds of pathomechanisms.

4.5 INFLAMMATION AND THE PRETERM BRAIN

Going back to the distinction between causal and conceptual pluralism, we now have to ask whether pathomechanistic pluralism refers to (1) fundamentally different kinds of real-life pathomechanistic processes that contribute to illness occurrence *qua* fundamentally different functions in the disease causation process, or (2) just fundamentally different kinds of pathomechanistic *concepts*.

In order to be able to endorse the notion that there are different kinds of pathomechanisms, not just different *concepts* of it, we need to show *how* different real-life pathomechanisms work. As an example, let me briefly outline the story of my own etiological research over the past 20 years. Aspects of my work will be aligned with Susser's *forms of determination* (causal production, predisposition, necessitation, and immanence). Moreover, two other forms of pathogenesis are added that come in the form of causal interaction (preconditioning and sensitization). For the sake of brevity, one paragraph is devoted to each of these plus the following, introductory paragraph that sets the stage.

Birth before the end of the normal gestation period of about 40 weeks is associated with a prominently increased risk for perinatal brain damage and subsequent neurodevelopmental disability (Pascal et al. 2018). The classic etiological model has been that lack of oxygen (hypoxia) and of cerebral blood flow (ischemia) damage the immature brain, leading to neurological disorders such as spastic cerebral palsy (du Plessis and Volpe 2002). My own work has focused on the observation that preterm birth is often a consequence of intrauterine infection, and on the hypothesis that inflammatory responses of the fetus and newborn might contribute to both the preterm birth process and the neurodevelopmental disabilities among preterm infants (Dammann and Leviton 1997, 2004). Along this line of thinking, circulating inflammatory proteins called *cytokines* play pivotal roles (Dammann and O'Shea 2008).

Inflammation-associated cytokines are proteins that are released by white blood cells in response to an infectious stimulus and which can *produce* tissue damage by leading to cell necrosis. One example is the cytokine tumor necrosis factor-alpha (TNF-α), which is capable of dissolving rapidly developing tumor tissue in mice (Old 1985). Administration of a closely related cytokine, interleukin 1-beta (IL-1β), to newborn mice results in brain damage and neurodevelopmental disability as seen in preterm human babies (Favrais et al. 2011).

Any gene mutation that leads to an increased production of pro-inflammatory cytokines should *predispose* a preterm infant to an increased risk of brain damage (Dammann, Durum, and Leviton 1999). This means that preterm infants who carry such genetic variants should be at increased risk for neurodevelopmental disabilities, which has been confirmed for genetic mutations that encode for increased production of TNF-α and IL-1β (Kapitanovic Vidak et al. 2012).

It is not difficult to find an example for what Susser calls a *precondition* (like male sex as a precondition for prostatic disease). Perhaps the most prominent precondition for inflammatory brain damage in preterm newborns is being born at a very early gestational age. This notion is far from trivial. Immaturity renders the brain more vulnerable to developmental insults, because the brain is exposed to adversity at earlier developmental stages, yielding more serious structural and functional changes compared to infants exposed to similar insults at later developmental stages. Brain damage etiology, neuropathology, and clinical appearance differ appreciably between preterm and term infants.

Susser's *immanence* is yet another kind of causation that comes "from the inside," so to speak. In this sense, developmental disabilities such as spastic cerebral palsy are immanent in children exposed to sustained perinatal inflammatory insult(s). In essence, the child proceeds along her "programmed" developmental trajectory after the perinatal insult, and disability emerges with development.[16]

One of the specific pathomechanisms we identified in our research is the *interaction* of risk factors in the form of double hits. One particular form is *preconditioning* (not to be confused with Susser's precondition as mentioned earlier), a situation where "a sub-injurious exposure renders the brain less vulnerable to a subsequent damaging exposure" (Hagberg et al. 2004). Another kind of double-hit situation occurs when the same kind of insult occurs twice, thereby exaggerating the damage. We observed this *sensitization* effect when prenatal (placenta) inflammation and postnatal inflammation co-occurred (Yanni et al. 2017). Of course, such interaction effects also occur when different kinds of preconditioners and sensitizers precede other insults (Eklind et al. 2005; Mallard and Hagberg 2007).

All kinds of pathomechanism reviewed in the preceding paragraphs are observable features of the etiological process of brain damage and subsequent neurodevelopment in preterm infants (or in animal models thereof). The references given, and many more in the perinatal neuroscience literature, summarize observations that support the notion that these pathogenetic mechanisms are real-world phenomena, not just concepts.

In this chapter, the idea of etiological explanations was reviewed from a pluralist perspective. The question of what part of the etiological process, if any, is plural was asked, and my answer is that we have both a pluralism of causes and a pluralism of causation before us. A variety of kinds of causes and kinds of causation were discussed, the latter in reference to an example from my own research. The conclusion is that etiological pluralism is real-life pluralism of both causes and causation of illness occurrence.

5 DIFFERENCE-MAKING AND MECHANISM

5.1 INTRODUCTION

In 2007, the author wrote with Alan Leviton that "[a]pparently, causal inference needs support from both observation and experiment, from both epidemiology and laboratory research" (Dammann and Leviton 2007). We also proposed four "criteria" that might support the claim that a certain risk factor might be causal: (1) the factor precedes damage, (2) it can produce damage in the experimental setting, (3) it is (statistically) associated with damage in (well-powered) observational studies, and (4) its absence from populations reduces the prevalence of damage compared to populations with the factor present. We saw the first as a requirement of causal primacy, the second as one of causal capability, the third as ascertaining that the problem is real, and the fourth as counterfactual, prospective manipulationist "proof of the pudding."

At around the same time, in 2007, Federica Russo and Jon Williamson published what is now known as the Russo–Williamson thesis (RWT). They observed that in the health sciences, causal claims are often supported by both evidence of difference-making (statistical associations) and evidence of mechanisms. Indeed, they went beyond this descriptive version of the RWT and stated a bit more prescriptively that "[t]o establish causal claims, scientists need the mutual support of mechanisms and dependencies" (Russo and Williamson 2007b).

In this chapter is offered an in-depth analysis of the RWT. First, an overview is provided of the papers by Russo and Williamson that proposed the RWT (Section 5.2). Second, criticism offered by others is discussed (Section 5.3). My own take is summarized in Section 5.3. My conclusion is that the RWT constitutes a descriptive account of the causation process that constitutes the first component of the etiological process, the substrate of etiological explanations.

5.2 RUSSO–WILLIAMSON THESIS

5.2.1 Mechanism and difference-making

In order to prevent illness, it is often sufficient to know the causes. Severing the connection between the causes of the causes and the causes themselves helps prevent the occurrence of illness. This is the application domain of public health. Severing the connection between the causes and illness occurrence requires knowledge about the pathogenetic mechanism. This is the domain of medicine. Thus, both public health and medical interventions need to be based on a detailed understanding of the process that leads to illness.

Between 2007 and 2011, Federica Russo and Jon Williamson published three papers that, taken together, established and elaborated on what is now known as the RWT (Russo 2009; Russo and Williamson 2007b, 2011b). In a nutshell, Russo and Williamson argue that "the health sciences make causal claims on the basis of evidence both of physical mechanisms, and of probabilistic dependencies" (Russo and Williamson 2007b).

Although it reads like a descriptive notion, some read the RWT as a normative/prescriptive statement,[1] as in "scientists *need* the mutual support of mechanisms and dependencies" (Russo and Williamson 2007b:159; emphasis mine). Russo has clarified that this normativity applies to knowledge gathering, not to health (care) activities: "RWT is prescriptive about what we should establish at the level of knowledge, not what we should do."[2]

The RWT has been extensively criticized.[3] Perhaps the heaviest blow so far comes from Joffe, who argues that "causation in the actual living world has to involve both mechanism and difference making, and that they play a complementary role" (Joffe 2013:180). Indeed, he calls this "not a plea for pluralism, that different accounts fit different situations, but rather an integrative-monist account in which these two key aspects are *necessarily* present" (p. 180; italics in original).

First, and most important in our context, is the idea that if the RWT is indeed mainly about the gathering of scientific knowledge about illness occurrence, it is not about two kinds of evidence used to support causal claims but about etiological explanations. The term *etiology* is used here as defined by MacMahon and Pugh (1970): a two-part sequence of causal events and subsequent pathogenetic mechanism. Traditionally, epidemiology is seen as dealing with the former, bench science with the latter.

Second, if the RWT is indeed about etiological explanations, difference-making and mechanism can be viewed as interrelated perspectives used to look at three kinds of evidence: exposure-outcome evidence that establishes the *why* of illness occurrence (causation – mainly in epidemiology), pathogenetic evidence that establishes the *how* of illness occurrence (pathogenesis – mainly in the lab), as well as the interventional evidence that confirms that our etiological explanation is correct (intervention – randomized controlled trial [RCT] in humans; experiments at the bench).

Third, Russo and Williamson might cast the net a bit too wide by referring to the "health sciences." They may be referring to not all the health sciences, but to the specific branches of science that perform illness occurrence research, that is, epidemiological research in human populations and basic bench research in animals or simpler systems.

In this book, the proposal is defended that mechanisms and dependencies are two closely related, nonindependent kinds of evidence used to study the process of illness causation. Therefore, the RWT may be correct, but trivially so, because mechanisms and difference-making *necessarily* co-occur, not only in support of causal claims but also in support of pathogenetic and confirmatory interventional claims. Whether we practice basic laboratory, epidemiological, or interventional research, we *always* rely on *both* evidence of mechanism and on difference-making, because all three approaches yield mechanistic *and* difference-making data.

5.2.2 Four papers promoting the Russo–Williamson thesis

Russo and Williamson have proposed and defended their thesis in a number of papers. In what follows is a summary of the most significant ones in establishing the RWT.

5.2.2.1 Interpreting causality in health sciences

In their first paper, Russo and Williamson begin by stating that the health sciences target two kinds of causes, that is, causes of disease and of effective treatment (Russo and Williamson 2007b:157). They state that health scientists have two goals, explanation and inference (ibid.), and argue, in explicit opposition to Lipton and Ødegaard (2005) that in order to intervene, it is insufficient to have evidence that exposure E is statistically associated with outcome O. Instead, they hold that one needs causal information *as well*. The authors provide examples from the health literature, stating that "[t]o establish causal claims, scientists need the mutual support of mechanisms and dependencies" (p. 159).

Russo and Williamson explain that by "probabilistic and mechanistic evidence" they refer to statistical correlations and biological changes at the microscopic level. They argue against both monist and pluralist accounts of causation in the health sciences, and conclude that neither account will do. Instead, they suggest that Williamson's proposed epistemic account of causation is a good third candidate.[4] With this account, Williamson proposes the view that

> the causal relation is mental rather than physical: a causal structure is part of an agent's representation of the world, just as a belief function is, and causal claims do not directly supervene on mind-independent features of the world. (Williamson 2005:130)

The main reason why Russo and Williamson think that epistemic causation provides a good backdrop for causation in the health sciences is because

> [I]n the health sciences it is clear that there are a variety of kinds of evidence. For example, in cancer science one might have a dataset containing clinical observations relating to past patients, another containing observations at the molecular level, some knowledge of the underlying biological mechanisms, some knowledge about the semantic relationships between variables provided by medical ontologies, and so on. All these types of evidence will shape causal beliefs about cancer: the datasets provide statistical evidence concerning difference-making; mechanisms provide evidence of stability; semantic relationships may provide evidence against causal connection (two dependent variables that are ontologically but not mechanistically related do not require a causal connection to account for their dependence). The epistemic theory of causality can account for this multi-faceted epistemology, since it deems the relationship between the various types of evidence and the ensuing causal claims to be constitutive of causality itself. Causality just *is* the result of this epistemology. On the other hand, a monistic account of causality in terms of just one of its indicators will

struggle to explain why the other indicators are so important. A pluralistic account will struggle to explain the apparent unity to our concept of cause and how any particular causal claim can have multi-faceted evidence. (Russo and Williamson 2007b:168; emphasis in original)

5.2.2.2 Generic versus single-case causality: The case of autopsy

In their second paper, Russo and Williamson turn to the distinction between generic/single-case causality, a kind of type/token distinction, as in "smoking causes lung cancer" versus "Harry's smoking caused his lung cancer" (Russo and Williamson 2011b). Their main question is how the generic and single-case levels are metaphysically related, and they offer three potential scenarios: either level is reducible to the other or "each level is to be analyzed individually" (p. 54). As an example from medicine, Russo and Williamson discuss in detail how causal inference is being handled in autopsy and argue that in *forensic* autopsy, "single-case non-causal evidence is used in conjunction with generic causal knowledge to establish a single-case causal claim" (p. 57) while in *academic* autopsy,

> single-case non-causal evidence is used in conjunction with generic knowledge of mechanisms, theoretical background knowledge and generic causal knowledge to establish single-case causal claims. But these single-case causal relations are then generalised by induction to a *new* generic causal claim. Academic autopsies thus contribute, unlike the other kinds of autopsy, to generic medical knowledge. (p. 58)

Based on this distinction, Russo and Williamson conclude that

> most metaphysical theories of causality—including pluralistic combinations of these theories—analyse any particular causal relation either in terms of difference-making relations or in terms of mechanistic relations, but not both. In the health sciences in general and in the case of autopsy in particular, evidence both of mechanisms and of difference-making is *normally* required to establish a causal claim. (pp. 61–2; emphasis mine)

Here, the authors modify their thesis by inserting the qualifier "normally"; they move away from their earlier, more rigid, and prescriptive version toward a more constrained realm of "normalcy." They also soften the initial version by stating that they had previously "put forward in Russo and Williamson (2007a,b) that *typically* evidence both of mechanisms and of difference-making is required to establish a causal claim" (p. 63; emphasis mine). In sum, it seems as if Russo and Williamson, in their second paper, felt the need to open a backdoor, allowing for cases where having evidence both of mechanisms and of difference-making is *not necessary* to establish causal claims. Using this exit route, they make it clear that they do *not* think that a "simple-minded conjunctive analysis" would do the job, simply because some known causal relations make a difference but have no mechanism, while others have a mechanism but make no difference (Williamson 2009).

As they did in their first paper, Russo and Williamson end their second with the proposal to tackle the "autopsy" problem with the epistemic account of causality. Here we go again:

The epistemic theory proceeds as follows. A causal epistemology can be thought of as a mapping from sets of possible evidence to sets of causal relationships: given one's evidence, a causal epistemology yields one or more sets of causal relationships that are compatible with that evidence. Now imagine that one had total evidence—one knew everything there was to know about the fundamental furniture of the world: the fundamental objects and the pattern of instantiation of the fundamental properties and the fundamental relations. Presumably, then, the correct causal epistemology— call it mapping ε—would yield the correct set of causal relationships. (This ought to be the case whatever one's metaphysical views about causality.) The epistemic theory takes this to be all there is to causality: according to this view, the causal relation is not one of the fundamental relations to be taken as basic in an ontology, nor does it supervene on the fundamental stuff by being definable in terms of difference-making or mechanisms; rather the correct set of causal relationships is just the set of relationships that would result from applying mapping ε to total evidence. The epistemic theory, then, analyses the causal relation in terms of causal epistemology. (p. 64)

Russo and Williamson hold that this view yields a metaphysical theory that is tightly linked with the epistemological theory, because "if causal relationships are what the epistemic theory says they are, there is no mystery as to how one can come to know about them" (p. 65). The epistemic theory treats both single-case and generic causal claims, and mechanistic and difference-making evidence on a par, thereby allowing for evidential pluralism while maintaining a metaphysical monist stance.

5.2.2.3 Epistemic causality and evidence-based medicine

In a companion paper published the same year, Russo and Williamson ask "what causal claims mean in the context of disease" (Russo and Williamson 2011a:563). The authors begin by stating that causal claims have become a rarity in biomedicine and that talk about correlations prevails. Again, they suggest that evidence of correlation is insufficient for intervention; instead, we need evidence of causation:

> Research papers in the biomedical sciences that draw conclusions about correlations are only of interest for diagnosis, prognosis, and treatment of diseases to the extent that those correlations are understood as supporting corresponding causal claims. (p. 563)

Nevertheless, they think that causal considerations have made it back into the biomedical sciences through the work of Peter Spirtes, Clark Glymour, and colleagues (1993) and Judea Pearl (2000) who, according to Russo and Williamson, have clarified the relationship between correlation and causation,[5] leading to a renaissance of causality in the biomedical sciences that deserves philosophical attention for at least two reasons. First, the distinction between generic and single-case causation needs to be explicated (which they do in the companion paper reviewed earlier). Second, it needs to be defined what we mean by claims like "A is a cause of B." They direct their attention to the second issue and state that what we mean is either that A makes a difference to B or that there is a mechanism connecting A and B. They then argue against this dual meaning claim, suggest an alternative interpretation from their epistemic perspective, and defend it. They end with a checklist of how all this would play out in what is called evidence-based medicine (EBM) (Group), a method developed in the 1990s to formally summarize results from multiple randomized intervention trials (Sackett and Rosenberg 1995). This concept, also known as meta-analysis, is widely used in biomedicine in order to generate a stronger evidence base for medical interventions than that provided by single randomized trials.

The authors' main point in applying the epistemic theory of causation to EBM has two parts. First, Russo and Williamson argue that the epistemic theory is the best, in fact the only fit for "causal assessment in medicine," referring to the Hill guidelines (Russo and Williamson 2011a:570). They "argue that an epistemic interpretation of causality is required to underpin Hill's causal assessment" (p. 571). Second, they move on to the "evidence hierarchy" in EBM, where the highest level of evidential authority is given to meta-analyses of RCTs, while expert opinion is at the lowest level. They criticize this hierarchy as (1) not being a hierarchy of evidence but of techniques of evidence-generation and (2) ignoring mechanistic evidence by looking for difference-making evidence only (at least at higher levels). Their declared main point here is that

> [S]ince the evidence hierarchy only really includes evidence of difference making (except perhaps at the bottom level, level IV), it loses the generality of Bradford Hill's guidelines for causal assessment, which treat mechanistic and difference-making evidence on an equal footing. (p. 573)

Again, Russo and Williamson's goal in this paper appears to be twofold: offer arguments in favor of the RWT and advertise the epistemic theory of causation.

5.2.2.4 EnviroGenomarkers

In yet another publication, Russo and Williamson discuss an example from recent research in biomedicine (Russo and Williamson 2012). They discuss the EnviroGenomarkers project, a scientific multipartner collaboration designed to elucidate the association between environmental exposures and disease. They describe the project as identifying biomarkers (genetic or protein markers in tissue or blood) of exposure and disease and generating *chains of difference-making*, and they argue that difference-making is *not* the only evidence that can be derived from the observational studies that the project is analyzing, because they agree with molecular epidemiologists who think that biomarkers can help establish causal pathways (Vineis and Perera 2007).

Before they explain their view of causation in the context of the EnviroGenomarkers project, Russo and Williamson ask whether evidence of mechanisms is enough to establish causal claims, and they argue that it is not. They distinguish between process-tracing (Salmon-Dowe) versus complex-systems mechanisms and suggest that "in order to capture the mechanisms of EnviroGenomarkers, one needs to appeal to both Salmon-Dowe processes and complex-system mechanisms" (p. 256).

Finally, we get a glimpse of what Russo and Williamson conceive as "disease causation":

> Yet, while the process leading from exposure to the body may resemble a Salmon-Dowe process, that is not the end of the story. Disease causation is much more complex than the one-off process leading from Billy throwing the stone at the bottle to its shattering. It usually takes many instances of exposure to cause disease — up to the moment in

which a threshold of "clinical vulnerability" is reached — and what goes on within the human body — involving the complex systems mechanisms for cell metabolism, cell repair, cell death and so on — very much determines whether and when disease will occur.

On the other hand, neither are these complex-systems mechanisms the end of the story. When the complex systems mechanisms for maintaining the integrity of the body fail, various processes are set in action that can lead ultimately to disease. These processes may be better understood as Salmon-Dowe processes than as mechanisms for disease, due to their unstable and irregular nature. Thus while one might perhaps say that a particular kind of cancer has a mechanism for tumour growth, it may be more natural to conceptualise a haemorrhage as a Salmon-Dowe process. (p. 257)

This quote suggests that Russo and Williamson use the term *disease causation* for the *entire* process from initial exposure to clinical disease occurrence. Most epidemiologists, however, acknowledge that they cannot speak to the issue of pathogenesis and tend to restrict the term *causation* to the causal role of observable risk factors that act as the initiators of the pathogenetic process.

5.3 ITS CRITICS

The RWT has been criticized from the biomedical (Gillies 2011), philosophical (Broadbent 2011; Illari 2011; Weber 2009), social science (Claveau 2012), and epidemiological perspective (Fiorentino and Dammann 2015). In this section, each criticism is briefly described without much comment and categories of objections are identified. In Section 5.4, a few thoughts that go beyond those categories are offered.

5.3.1 Weber

Erik Weber agrees with the RWT in that he subscribes to an evidential pluralist perspective (using evidence of difference-making *and* of mechanism) and to an output monist view that assumes that health scientists use only one single notion of cause. His main argument is the one indicated in his article's title that probabilistic theories of causation can account for the use of mechanistic evidence. My main problem with this hypothesis is that its formulation makes it hard to grasp what the author means. "To account for" usually means "to explain."[6] Thus translated, one way to read Weber's hypothesis is that *working in a probabilistic framework can explain why mechanistic evidence is used*. Another meaning – "to account for" as meaning "to be a particular amount or part of something" – does not make sense in this context.

Weber reviews one particular probabilistic theory[7] and suggests that this theory is superior to other probabilistic theories (those of Suppes, Eels, and Humphreys) because it "defines causation in terms of what would happen in hypothetical populations, [while] those of Suppes, Eells, and Humphreys [,] define causation in terms of probabilistic relations in the real world." This statement suggests that Weber prefers the potential outcomes approach to causation[8] over others, which he confirms in a footnote, where he writes that others have used "a 'potential outcome model' of causation" (Weber 2009:293). His argument boils down to the notion that using mechanistic evidence is rational because

> it happens that we want to make causal claims about populations while no probabilistic evidence is available. [...] in such cases, mechanistic evidence can help: a bottom-up argument [...] can lead to conclusions about the hypothetical populations X and K. It cannot give us a precise estimate of PX(E) and PK(E). However, [...] this is not a problem: all we need is an argument that PX(E) is different from PK(E) [...] for a historian or social scientist that wants to make a Gierean causal claim about a population, it is perfectly rational to gather mechanistic evidence, since that evidence can help him to establish the claim. (p. 286)

Weber concludes that "[t]his undermines the thesis of Russo and Williamson that probabilistic theories of causality cannot account for the use of mechanistic evidence" (p. 293).

5.3.2 Gillies: Reformulation

Donald Gillies suggests a reformulation of the RWT because he thinks that two distinctions need to be appreciated (Gillies 2011). First, he suggests that in the health sciences, the evidence of difference-making and of mechanism are represented by evidence from observational epidemiology and experimental laboratory research, respectively. Second, he suggests that the RWT comes in a strong and a weak form, depending on whether a mechanism is confirmed or plausible, respectively. He prefers this weak version:

> In order to establish that A causes B, observational statistical evidence does not suffice. Such evidence needs to be supplemented by interventional evidence, which can take the form of showing that there is a plausible mechanism linking A to B. (p. 115)

5.3.3 Illari: Disambiguation

This, of course, opens an entirely new can of worms: is the RWT about causal evidence or about evidence of causation, and about mechanistic evidence or evidence of mechanism? Phyllis Illari has argued that the RWT "is multiply ambiguous, so that it has a range of possible interpretations" (Illari 2011:140). Her first major point is that Russo and Williamson do not write about ways of mechanistic evidence generation, but about evidence of mechanisms and difference making. She argues that both, the evidence gathering techniques on the one hand and types of evidence on the other, are independent. She thinks that "there is no particular reason to assume, in advance of investigation, that any particular evidence-gathering method can only be used to gather evidence of one particular type of thing" (p. 141).

This author completely agrees with Illari that, for example, results from laboratory experiments need first to be difference-making to be counted as mechanistic evidence and that observations of difference-making (associations between risk factors and health outcomes) can indeed provide mechanistic evidence even outside the realm of RCTs, for example, via data manipulation.

5.3.4 Broadbent: Usefulness without mechanism

Alex Broadbent argues that the RWT is mistaken in its normative form, which states that in order to establish a causal claim, the identification of an underlying mechanism is necessary, but not sufficient, because statistical evidence is needed as well (Broadbent 2011:57). Instead, Broadbent argues that knowledge about the underlying mechanism is not necessary for a health intervention to be practically useful (p. 68).

Broadbent holds that epidemiologists do not need evidence of mechanisms but can initiate *successful* interventions based only on evidence of difference-making.[9] For example, he writes that the RWT would justify the stance that, if the germ theory was not yet accepted, it would be rational not to accept Semmelweis' life-saving intervention (require medical students and physicians to wash their hands after they have finished working in the morgue and before they attend to their patients in the maternity ward), "no matter how much evidence we had gathered in the meantime about the efficacy if disinfecting hands" (pp. 58–9). He concludes that "refusing to make a causal inference until a mechanism is known can be seriously detrimental to public health" (p. 60).

Broadbent goes further and rejects the RWT even in its descriptive form, because there are definitely instances in which it just is not the case that causal claims in the health sciences are based on both evidence of difference-making *and* evidence of mechanisms. Indeed, the Semmelweis case as presented is such an instance in which no mechanistic evidence was available to support the causal claim other than his assumption that "the cause of the greater mortality rate was cadaverous particles adhering to the hands of examining obstetricians. I removed this cause by chlorine washings. Consequently, mortality in the first clinic fell below that of the second" (Semmelweis 1983).

Russo and Williamson respond directly to this concern in their third paper on the RWT, where they state that their argument was that "in the health sciences, it is a matter of fact that mechanistic and difference-making evidence are treated in an egalitarian way when establishing causal claims" (Russo and Williamson 2011a:576). They call this their "descriptive claim," which may be immune to Broadbent's objection not because Broadbent is wrong, but because Russo and Williamson have shifted the goalposts sideways ever so gently. They also "advocate the strong normative thesis that […] one ought to treat mechanistic and difference-making evidence in an egalitarian way" (p. 576). Again, this is a lateral move that helps them evade Broadbent's criticism without responding to it. Egalitarian necessity to justify causal claims was what they requested in their earlier papers, not egalitarian treatment. Thus, I think that Broadbent's point still stands unrefuted.

5.3.5 Claveau: Two theses

François Claveau sees the RWT as two theses, not one (Claveau 2012). In his view,

> the first Russo–Williamson Thesis is that a causal claim can only be established when it is jointly supported by difference-making and mechanistic evidence. ... The second [...] is that standard accounts of causality fail to handle the dualist epistemology highlighted in the first Thesis. (p. 806)

However, instead of elevating Claveau's second RWT to the status of "Thesis," in this book it is considered a mere characteristic of the first. Thus, RWT is used in the singular.

Claveau objects to the first by describing a counterexample that has established causation based on mechanistic evidence only, and to the second by arguing that the counterfactual-manipulationist account of causation "can make perfect sense of the typical strategy in [his] case study to draw on both difference-making and mechanistic evidence." In the biomedical health sciences, both correlative, difference-making and mechanistic evidence are part of both epidemiological studies and experimental bench research. This may all be "just an instance of the common strategy of increasing evidential variety" (p. 812). However, the four types of evidence defined by cross-tabulating these two dyads do not just increase evidential variety in the qualitative sense by gathering support for a causal hypothesis from various different angles, but also in the sense of strengthening our justification of that causal claim, which moves from weaker to stronger on a fictitious evidential scale with each additional piece of evidence we accumulate.

5.4 MY TAKE

Russo and Williamson fail to give solid arguments for their descriptive and normative claims (Section 5.4.1); they leave unclear what they mean by "the health sciences," and "disease causation" differs from scientific definitions (Section 5.4.2); and they are imprecise in what kind of evidence of mechanism the RWT requires (Section 5.4.3). My view is that difference-making is causal by definition (Section 5.4.4) and explains how mechanisms can be different in three ways, distinguishing between entity-based, association-based, and activity-based mechanistic evidence (Section 5.4.5). If the RWT is true, it might be truism (Section 5.4.6).

5.4.1 Where is the argument?

The RWT is a simple description of what "health scientists" have always done: they mount evidence in support of a causal hypothesis by drawing on all kinds of evidence. Russo and Williamson acknowledge that Hill's nine "viewpoints" do exactly that, that is, strengthen causal claims. In support, they quote Kundi: "the Bradford Hill criteria were established such that, in the case they are met for a specific factor, this would increase our confidence in this factor being causally related to the disease" (Kundi 2006:970). They do not make an argument. All they do is use their observation of dual usage as support for the "need-both argument," which it cannot provide. Just because both are used does not implicate that both *have to be* used. Thus, although the authors cogently demonstrate that the evidential dyad they champion is used in causal inference in epidemiology and medicine, merely showing that evidence of both difference-making and mechanism *is used* to support causal claims does not at all support the notion that they *are necessary* to support causal claims. One response to this objection would be that the "observation of dual usage" was not intended to support the need-both argument; it was just stated as a fact that usage of both can be observed when looking at professional practice, preempting possible objections that would arise if we could *not* make such observation. This response, however, would not contradict my claim; it would just inform us that Russo and Williamson brought it up as some kind of background information for their need-both argument.

A more intriguing response, and actually the one that Russo and Williamson seem to advance, would be the claim that "observation of dual usage" does indeed support the need-both argument, because the "observation of dual usage" somehow *depends* on the truth of the need-both argument. In other words, the response would mount a counterfactual argument along the lines of "If the need-both argument were false, dual usage could not be observed." This response, however, fails because it is eminently obvious that dual usage can be observed regardless of whether we always need just one or both kinds of evidence. For example, nowhere do the "Hill guidelines" require that all nine need to be checked off to support a causal claim. Rather, as eminent pediatrician and epidemiologist Leon Gordis states, "it is not so much a count of the number of guidelines present that it is relevant to causal inference but rather an *assessment of the total pattern of evidence observed* that may be consistent with one or more of the guidelines" (Gordis 2014:253; italics in original). Thus, the fact that both kinds of evidence are reflected in the Hill guidelines does not suffice to support the need-both argument because it could certainly be the case that a causal claim finds support by only "one or more of the guidelines," which may or may not include guidelines representing both kinds of evidence.

5.4.2 What are "the health sciences" and "disease causation?"

Broadbent's critique of the RWT (as outlined earlier) invalidates the RWT by showing that it is too broad. Broadbent talks about epidemiology and public health; Russo and Williamson talk about the health sciences. Unfortunately, Russo and Williamson do not really tell us what they mean by "the health sciences." The term is only vaguely defined in Russo and Williamson's papers; it is unclear if pharmacology and medicine, as well as epidemiology and public health would count as health sciences. Thus, the thought is (in accordance with Broadbent) that the RWT might have some value *in some but not all* of the health sciences, and certainly not in epidemiology and public health.

While Broadbent's example of intervention being justified without knowledge of mechanisms is certainly true in epidemiology and public health, it is not true in pharmacology and medicine. Here, knowledge of mechanisms is of crucial importance because pharmacological interventions are designed to interfere with pathomechanisms.

But here, the two kinds of evidence support two different kinds of causal claims: the mechanistic evidence from pharmacological research supports the claim that pathomechanism P_1 does indeed cause a certain disease, while the difference-making evidence from RCT supports the claim that the drug works. However, it could also be the case that the drug does *not* interfere with P_1 but instead with a completely separate pathomechanism P_2 that also leads to the disease of interest.

5.4.3 Evidence of what kind of mechanism?

Russo and Williamson do not specify in much detail what kinds of mechanisms they refer to. It seems as if they mean biological, a.k.a., pathogenetic mechanisms, sometimes called *causal pathways*. Vineis and Perera (2007) claim that biomarkers can help establish causal pathways. In such research, biological molecular markers of pathogenetic processes are measured in epidemiological studies and analyzed in the same way risk factors are analyzed, that is, by relying on biostatistical evidence of difference-making. Still, molecular biomarker epidemiologists claim that knowledge of biomarkers can provide insight into the mechanism of action: "molecular epidemiology approaches facilitate testing the association between mechanistic events in a defined continuum" (Schulte and Perera 1993:7). From this perspective, molecular epidemiology helps elucidate pathomechanisms by finding associations between components, which is evidence of difference-making. Thus, at least in the context of biomarker epidemiology, evidence of difference-making is used to establish evidence of mechanism.

5.4.4 Difference-*making*?

Initially, Russo and Williamson used the term "probabilistic dependence" to denote their view that "a cause needs to make a difference to its effects, that is, there needs to be some appropriate probabilistic dependence" (Russo and Williamson 2007b:159). Later, they replace "probabilistic dependence" with "difference-making," because "causes are difference-makers" (Russo 2009), which is in keeping with the view of both philosophers of science (Bunge 1979) and epidemiologists (MacMahon and Pugh 1970; Susser 1991). In probabilistic theories of causality, such difference generated by a cause is an increased probability of its effect to occur (Eells 1991). Russo takes this definition and runs with it: "We will know about causes of disease by investigating whether some specific variations in exposure lead to variations in disease," and states that "the definitions of cause are underpinned by a variational epistemology" (Russo 2009:544).

First, *difference-making* is not a good term for evidence based on quantitative relationships such as associations and correlations *that may or may not be causal*. Difference-*making* suggests that the difference is indeed *made*, which in turn bears causal meaning, thus making the claim circular and a noninformative "explanation." The same goes for "dependencies"; *dependence* suggests a causal link. But if *all* difference-making is causal, why is difference-making evidence alone insufficient to support a causal claim?

Second, difference-making is not separate from evidence of mechanism. Difference-making evidence is used to establish exposure-outcome evidence (e.g., in epidemiological studies) and to elucidate mechanisms (e.g., in biological bench experiments).

5.4.5 Three kinds of evidence

In our discussion of the RWT's difference-making and mechanism in the context of evidence-based medicine, the suggestion is to replace, at least in the health sciences, "evidence of difference-making" or "evidence of dependencies" by the less causally fraught term "exposure-outcome evidence," honoring the epidemiological terminology for the purported cause-effect relationship (Fiorentino and Dammann 2015). More importantly, however, we suggest a more detailed appreciation of what constitutes evidence of mechanism.

In particular, we advocate a view that distinguishes between entity-based, association-based, and activity-based mechanistic evidence, each one having a different explanatory power, according to complexity and context. Entity-based evidence is evidence of the presence and/or location of defined entities in a mechanism. For example, consider the following discovery of the presence of a certain signaling molecule:

> Fetal lung surfactant synthesis requires communication between mesenchyme and adjacent type II epithelial cells. The specific nature of the communication is poorly understood. Conditioned media from fetal lung fibroblasts stimulate fetal type II epithelial cells to synthesize surfactant. This activity is ascribed to the presence of an unidentified polypeptide, termed fibroblast–pneumocyte factor (FPF). Here we demonstrate that NRG-1, a stromal-derived growth factor active in cell–cell communication in mammary development, is secreted by fetal lung fibroblasts. Purified NRG-1β mimics the stimulatory effect of lung fibroblast-conditioned medium (FCM) on surfactant synbook. Moreover, a neutralizing antibody to NRG-1 inhibits this stimulatory activity in the FCM. This indicates that NRG-1β plays a major role in type II cell maturation. (Dammann, Nielsen, and Carraway 2003)

Association-based mechanistic evidence is, just like exposure outcome evidence, evidence of a statistical association between two phenomena. The only difference is that epidemiological exposure-outcome evidence describes such associations in human populations, while association-based mechanistic evidence describes associations of parts of mechanisms with one another. Activity-based evidence is direct evidence of activities (processes) in which parts of mechanisms are involved.

5.4.6 Is RWT a truism?

The RWT in its descriptive form ("causal claims in the health sciences receive support by both evidence of difference-making and evidence of mechanism") is an astute observation, but it lacks novelty. Russo and Williamson dissect the most frequently cited list of purported causal characteristics of epidemiological studies, Hill's guidelines, and separate them into characteristics of difference-making and

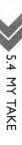

mechanism (Russo and Williamson 2007b). Thus, if the RWT is true, it is not new. Both kinds of evidence, mechanism and difference-making, are already on Hill's list, and both are often observed together.

Let us assume causation is really out there; a relation between two occurrences, of cause and effect, and that, at least in the health sciences (however defined), there is indeed a physical or biochemical process in between the two. In other words, let us assume that all causation in the health sciences needs a mechanism. In this case, evidence of mechanism, however generated or produced, would support a causal claim. Now the question is: do we need, as the RWT suggests, additional evidence of difference-making? There really is no choice, because *evidence of mechanism is also evidence of difference-making.*

It can be argued that the RWT may get it right, but only trivially so, because *all* evidence of causation in biomedicine is both difference-making *and* mechanistic. *Any* health-related causal phenomenon can be observed only by observing a difference, between exposed/intervention group and a control group, in *all* of analytical epidemiology and experimental bench science. Such differences can only be produced by mechanisms, biopsychosocial mechanisms at the population and individual levels. Observation of a difference (at the population level) suggests the presence of a mechanism at the level of the individual. The mechanism is what makes the difference, and the workings of the mechanism can only be elucidated by observing differences within the mechanism.

My somewhat provocative argument would go as follows. All causation is mechanistic. All evidence in support of causal claims, therefore, *somehow* refers to mechanisms. Thus, all causal evidence is evidence of mechanism, and some evidence of difference-making is always part of evidence of mechanism. When we talk about causation we often mean to indicate that there is a mechanism that connects cause and effect. First, we have the differences made *in* the mechanism, among its parts, for example, the changes in relative position of the wheels and pinions in a clock movement). Second, we have the difference made *by* the mechanism, that is, the difference the mechanism makes between potential effects. However, this evidence is generated in different ways, using different perspectives or lenses, including the observation of difference-making under various conditions.

In this view, *evidence of mechanism and evidence of difference-making always coexist in causal explanations.* No causation without mechanism, no mechanism without difference-making. The observable difference-making inside the mechanism is evidence of a mechanism, while the observable difference between cause and effect is the result of (made by) that mechanism at work. While the former kind of evidence refers to causal relationships within the mechanism at a lower level, the latter refers to causal relationships that result from the mechanism at a higher level. Thus, evidence of mechanism boils down to observation of difference-making inside the mechanism, the difference being the changes in position and movement of the parts of the clockwork, while the "making" in this kind of difference-making is the constant provision of a driving force, the spring of the clock, another mechanism, even further down, which can only be established by observing further differences further down. It is impossible to observe the occurrence of the effect without observing a change in circumstances, that is, a difference. It is also impossible to gather evidence of mechanism without observing a difference. In essence, mechanisms make differences at a higher level; thus, higher-level difference-making is evidence for *the presence* of a mechanism. Lower-level difference-making is evidence for the mechanistics of the mechanism. One upshot of this proposal is that causation *just is* mechanisms at work, but this claim needs to be further explored.

In the health sciences, at least in those parts of the health sciences that concern themselves with illness causation, higher-level difference-making is observed at the level of the individual, in cases and case series by clinicians, and in larger study populations by epidemiologists. Lower-level difference-making is observed by bench scientists, who typically cannot wait until a mechanism pops up to be observed; thus, bench scientists generate models of disease that can be tested in the lab. Clinicians, epidemiologists, and bench scientists basically sandwich the mechanism by gathering difference-making evidence. In etiological explanations, the name for that mechanism is "pathomechanism."[10]

5.4.7 Support, not explanation?

Argument has been presented that while both kinds of evidence may *support* causal claims, they do not both *explain* a causal relationship. Instead, evidence of mechanistic function (lower-level difference-making) explains the causal claim, which in turn explains why we can observe exposure-outcome evidence (higher-level difference-making). We wrote that

> exposure-outcome evidence (previously known as difference-making evidence) provides associations that can be explained through a hypothesis of causation, while mechanistic evidence provides finer-grained associations and knowledge of entities that ultimately explains a causal hypothesis. (Fiorentino and Dammann 2015)

In essence, we accepted Broadbent's suggestion to shift from a focus on causation and causal inference to explanation and prediction (Broadbent 2013:8). We suggest that association-based mechanistic evidence [exposure – $x - y$ – outcome] is explained by a mechanistic causal claim [exposure $> x > y >$ outcome], which in turn explains the overall causal claim [exposure $>$ outcome].

In other words, could it be that the mechanism *just is* the causal process, and what the mechanism does *just is* what we mean by "causation"? If that is the case, we can amend our proposal quoted earlier to read

> Observations of the difference made by the occurrence of *the results* of mechanisms at work (e-o-evidence) can be explained through a hypothesis of causation (the hypothesis that there is a mechanism), while observations of the difference made by parts of the mechanism at work provide finer-grained associations and knowledge of entities that ultimately explains a causal hypothesis.

The current practice in the health sciences, broadly construed, goes beyond the RWT type of evidence. Difference-making and mechanistic types of evidence are *formal* types, classified by their respective roles as criteria for causal inference. In biomedicine, we need to consider *subject matter* types of evidence, of etiology (risk factors that might be causes) and pathogenesis (the biological disease mechanism).

Russo and Williamson appear to confuse these levels when they talk about probabilistic evidence as "observed dependencies in a range of similar studies" (Russo and Williamson 2007b:162) and about mechanistic evidence as "chemical reactions, electric signals, alterations at the cellular level, etc" (ibid.), respectively.

Russo and Williamson talk about two types of evidence and state that association (difference-making) and mechanism *support* single causal claims. Etiological explanations are different in that they consist of causes and pathomechanisms; they explain illness occurrence by referring to *which factors* contribute to the etiological process and *how*.

In keeping with this idea, it might be helpful to modify RWT and Illari's disambiguation in the context of illness occurrence:

> For illness occurrence to be explained comprehensively, we need evidence of both difference-making and of mechanism at both the exposure-outcome level and at the pathogenetic level, as evidence of the presence and function, respectively, of an etiological process.

Although this statement reads like a normative one, which it was claimed not to be prior to the RWT, my statement does not ask you to accept it for all etiological explanations, only for *comprehensive ones*. This is not a loophole to escape criticism but an acknowledgement that etiological explanations come in degrees. A causal explanation may refer to the causes of illness without reference to mechanisms, as in "excessive radiation causes skin cancer." Similarly, a mechanistic explanation may focus on mechanisms, without referring to causes, as in "impaired double-strand DNA breakage repair mechanisms lead to skin cancer." Both causal and mechanistic explanations can be considered *partial etiological explanations*. The RWT, conversely, does not provide evidence that comes in degrees, and it does not allow for partial conclusions that partially support causal claims. In etiological explanations, when causal explanations and mechanistic explanations come together to form causal-mechanical explanations, they become *comprehensive* and, thereby, *better* etiological explanations, in particular if they biologically plausibly enhance and support each other, and perhaps even fit coherently with other kinds of explanation into a unified etiological framework, which, for example, allows for multiple different etiological explanations for individual diseases or disorders.[11]

The concept of *mechanism* features prominently in the RWT and critiques thereof. Due to space limitations, a full-fledged critique of the current wave of thought about *mechanisms* in the philosophy of the health sciences is not presented (Broadbent 2011; Craver and Darden 2013; Williamson 2011a, 2011b). However, in this and the next chapter, it is argued that it would be worthwhile, at least in the context of etiological explanations, to at least consider a *process* view along with the focus on mechanisms. In the next chapter, this proposal is taken to the next level by zooming in on the idea that when we say that *X* causes *Y*, we not only imply that they are linked by a mechanism, we also imply that this mechanism is a *process*. Making both a bit more explicit might help make etiological explanations more useful.

6
PROCESS PERSPECTIVE

6.1 INTRODUCTION

In Chapter 5, the emphasis was on mechanisms as part of the Russo–Williamson thesis (RWT), which holds that causal claims in the health sciences require both evidence of difference-making and of mechanism. Agreement was made with Broadbent that RWT evidence is not necessary and not even universal in biomedical and population health practice for making causal claims (Broadbent 2011). Another difficulty with the RWT is that all difference-making must come with some mechanism that explains how the difference is made, and that mechanistic evidence always requires the observation of difference-making. On this view, the mechanism comes with implicit difference-making, and the observation of difference-making comes with implicit mechanism. Therefore, it was suggested to zoom in on *exposure-outcome* evidence, the high-level difference-making observed regarding differential outcomes in exposed versus nonexposed groups of individuals (Fiorentino and Dammann 2015). This kind of observation ("exposure is associated with the outcome") can be explained by a causal hypothesis ("exposure causes the outcome"), which in turn can be explained by pathomechanistic evidence ("mechanism M plausibly connects exposure and outcome"), which includes the observation of lower-level difference-making.

The focus in this chapter is on the *process perspective* of mechanism and etiological explanations. Why process? One reason is, at least in my thinking, that etiological explanations do more than RWT-like justifications of causal claims, precisely because they take a process view of what happens along the biological trajectory from cause to illness.[1]

First, they provide information about the *causation process* by proposing candidate causes and the pathomechanisms they initiate. Second, they provide information about the *disease process* by specifying how the pathomechanism leads to clinical illness. Third, they thus generate knowledge about the overarching *etiological process*.[2] For example, one possible etiological explanation of skin cancer would provide information about radiation and how it induces DNA double-strand breakage, specify how DNA double-strand breakage leads to uncontrolled skin cell growth and clinically visible skin abnormalities, and thereby generate knowledge about the overarching etiological *process* from radiation to skin cancer. Viewed from this perspective, talk about mechanism tells only part of the story, while talk about process tells the whole story (or at least more of it).

Another reason to take the process perspective is that a sole focus on causes would ignore the mechanism, and a sole focus on mechanism would ignore causes. Ignoring the mechanism may be acceptable in primary prevention, because a reduction in exposure should lead to a reduction in outcome at the population level, regardless of the mechanism. In medicine, however, knowledge of the pathomechanism is helpful for the development of pharmacological interventions. However, ignoring the causes in favor of the mechanism can lead to an inappropriate focus on details of purported mechanisms that generate unfruitful research. In the context of my own research field of perinatal neuroepidemiology, this has happened following initial reports from the 1960s that "trouble breathing" among newborns was causally responsible for the brain damage they sustained (Banker and Larroche 1962). Subsequent work focused almost exclusively on one purported pathomechanism, hypoxia-ischemia (Vannucci and Hagberg 2004), despite ample evidence that this mechanism is but one among multiple, and perhaps not even the most important pathomechanism (Gilles et al. 2017).

Section 6.2 is based on a paper previously published in the journal *Perspectives in Biology and Medicine* (Erdei and Dammann 2014).[3] In it, we mount the evidence in support of the notion that autism is not a static disorder but a process. We begin with a discussion of the unique link between preterm birth (birth before 37 weeks' gestational age) and autism. We then outline the link between immune system characteristics and both prematurity and autism. Finally, we suggest that Rothman's model of sufficient cause and component causes, combined with theories of causation concepts, can be interpreted as a mechanistic model of autism causation. In Section 6.3, clarification is made of some of the terminology we used in that paper by aligning it with the terminology used in this book. Differences and similarities between the ideas of mechanism and process in the context of etiology are presented.

6.2 PROCESS ETIOLOGY OF AUTISM[4]

6.2.1 Introduction

Explaining the causal mechanisms that contribute to autism spectrum disorder (ASD; henceforth, *autism*) occurrence remains a conundrum in developmental medicine, neuroscience, and child psychiatry (Ashwood et al. 2011; Goyal and Miyan 2014; Patterson 2009; Ronemus et al. 2014). Recent research has led to consensus about behavioral definitions and their underlying cognitive processes, early diagnosis and standardized assessments, evidence-based interventions, systems-level approaches to neurobiology, and identification of genetic variants and their interaction with epigenetic and environmental factors (Lai, Lombardo, and Baron-Cohen 2014). However, an *explanatory* model of autism causation remains elusive.

Perhaps, as suggested, it might be "time to give up on a single explanation for autism" (Happé, Ronald, and Plomin 2006) and, one might add, for other neurodevelopmental disorders as well, including, but not limited to, cerebral palsy, intellectual disability, or attention deficit hyperactivity disorder. Most experts will agree that autism occurrence is what has been called "multifactorial," in the sense that multiple factors play a role in it (Goyal and Miyan 2014; Hallmayer et al. 2011). Multiple individual risk factors have been proposed as possibly leading to autism, including genetic factors, *de novo* mutations, drug and environmental exposures, maternal infections during pregnancy, selenoenzymes and antioxidant metabolism, maternal nutrients and supplement deficiencies, or abnormalities in the gut flora (Atladottir et al. 2012; Braun et al. 2014; Gidaya et al. 2014; Gorrindo et al. 2012; Hallmayer et al. 2011; Iossifov et al. 2014; Lyall, Schmidt, and Hertz-Picciotto 2014; Raymond, Deth, and Ralston 2014; Ronemus et al. 2014; Sandin et al. 2014). Particular attention has been given in recent years to immune dysfunctions and neuro-inflammation as a common thread of some of these individual factors (Ashwood et al. 2011; Goyal and Miyan 2014; Meyer, Feldon, and Dammann 2011; Rossignol and Frye 2012).

6.2.2 Prematurity and autism

The question "What causes preterm birth?" has preoccupied researchers for decades (Bezold et al. 2013). At over 11%, the United States continues to have one of the highest rates of preterm birth among developed countries (Beck et al. 2010; Martin, Hamilton, and Osterman 2014). The idea put forward in this chapter is that whatever initiates the preterm birth process might also initiate abnormal pathways of brain development, thereby creating a "perfect storm" of interactions among genetic background and environmental exposures that initiates a fetal immune response and leads to both preterm birth and altered development of the brain and neural connectivity. It is possible that the ongoing process of inflammation, via activation of microglia, will ultimately result in what has been termed *encephalopathy of prematurity* (Volpe 2009), which in turn could lead to atypical neurodevelopment, including autism (Figure 6.1).

Many studies have reported an association between preterm birth and autism (Hack et al. 2009; Johnson et al. 2010; Kuban et al. 2009; Lampi et al. 2012; Limperopoulos

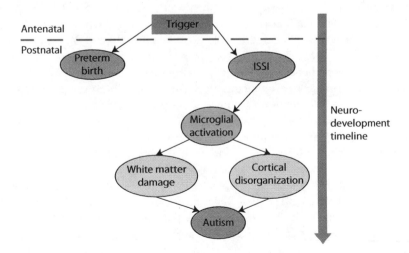

Figure 6.1 Inflammation, preterm birth, and autism causation. The initial trigger that occurs *in utero* can contribute to birth prior to term, and, at the same time, interferes with normal brain development and synapse formation mainly via microglial activation. This, in time, will lead to clinical features consistent with autism.

et al. 2008; Mahoney et al. 2013; Schendel and Bhasin 2008). One hypothesis that explains this association is that a sustained presence of inflammatory mediators in the maternal, fetal, and neonatal blood may not only initiate the preterm labor and delivery process but also interfere with normal brain development and increase a child's risk for atypical development (Dammann, Kuban, and Leviton 2002; Favrais et al. 2011; Malaeb and Dammann 2009; Meyer, Feldon, and Dammann 2011).

Cytokines and chemokines are inflammatory blood components present in the maternal, placental, and fetal compartments during pregnancy (Dammann and Leviton 1997). These proteins recruit cells to defend and repair the brain, but they sometimes also contribute to clinical disease (Jaffer, Wade, and Gourlay 2010). Importantly, these inflammatory proteins can act as the contributors to neurological and behavioral abnormalities (Dammann and O'Shea 2008; Kerschensteiner, Meinl, and Hohlfeld 2009). Animal and human studies suggest that inflammatory protein imbalances during critical windows in early brain development have the ability to sensitize the brain for subsequent insults (Aden et al. 2010; Du et al. 2011; Hagberg, Gressens, and Mallard 2012; Rousset et al. 2006; van de Looij et al. 2012). A major observation in autism research is the presence of inflammatory markers in the brain tissue or cerebrospinal fluid of individuals with autism (Morgan et al. 2010; Rodriguez and Kern 2011; Vargas et al. 2005; Zimmerman et al. 2005). Activation of microglia, a type of glial cell within the central nervous system involved in synaptogenesis, is one pivotal mechanism in the neuro-inflammatory process, and it may lead to alteration or even loss of neuronal connections (Chez et al. 2007; Li et al. 2005; Morgan et al. 2010; Rodriguez and Kern 2011; Vargas et al. 2005; Verney et al. 2012; Zimmerman et al. 2005). This altered connectivity may be due to the loss of neurons, whose migration toward the future cortical layers is interrupted by the "minefield" of activated microglia in the intermediate zone (future white matter) of the developing brain (Leviton and Gressens 2007). Many studies report altered brain connectivity in individuals with autism, and the degree of abnormalities in brain connectivity appears to be proportional to the severity of a child's behavioral symptoms (Barttfeld et al. 2011; Damarla et al. 2010; Di Martino et al. 2011; Just et al. 2012; Minshew and Keller 2010; Zikopoulos and Barbas 2013). In sum, neuro-inflammation, via cellular processes such as microglial activation, seems to play a central role in the pathogenesis of autism (Figure 6.1).

Children born preterm are one unique subset among individuals with autism. Their exposure to inflammation begins during pregnancy and can continue into the neonatal period and affect brain connectivity over long stretches in time. For example, systemic upregulation of pro-inflammatory cytokines is more common and more prominent in school-age children with cerebral palsy than in controls (Lin et al. 2010). As the systemic inflammation can be either intermittent or sustained, the term *intermittent or sustained systemic inflammation* (ISSI) has been proposed (Dammann and Leviton 2014). Since ISSI is linked to brain abnormalities in preterm newborns and prematurity is associated with autism, it follows that ISSI might be linked to autism in children born preterm. One crucial component of this causation-process model is that neuro-inflammation does not occur at a single point in time but rather constitutes an ongoing exposure during an individual's developmental trajectory (Malaeb and Dammann 2009). An ongoing interaction between innate and adaptive immune factors and the typical developmental process leads to

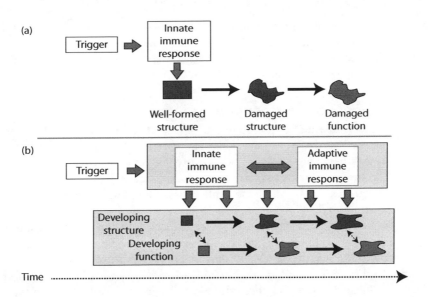

Figure 6.2 The traditional scenario of perinatal brain injury (a) postulates that a single and rather short insult damages existing structure and leads to altered function. The alternative view (b), postulates that after an initial trigger has occurred, an ongoing interaction between innate and adaptive immune processes adversely affects the development of brain structure and function over an extended time period. (Reproduced with permission from Malaeb, S. and O. Dammann. 2009. *J Child Neurol.* 24(9), 1119–26.)

immature brain structure changes, such as white matter abnormalities and neuronal/axonal deficits in the cortex, thalamus, basal ganglia, brainstem, and cerebellum. This, in turn, leads to altered neuronal connectivity, which underlies a spectrum of neurodevelopmental disorders, including autism, cerebral palsy, or intellectual disability, and it will lead to different abnormal function at different time points during development (Figure 6.2).

Understanding inflammatory causes and mechanisms in autism will provide clues about possible therapeutic strategies. One proposed hypothesis is that reducing the neurotoxic aspects of microglial activation might reduce the neurodestructive effects of chronic inflammation and allow for improvement of neuronal connectivity (Rodriguez and Kern 2011). To what degree such an approach might help improve behavioral symptoms at a clinical level is still a matter of speculation.

6.2.3 Causal-process model of autism

Evidence suggests that autism might not be a static disorder but a neuro-immunological process that interferes with another process, that of typical neurodevelopment. Both processes appear to contribute to the occurrence of autism, albeit in different ways. Therefore, both should be considered of etiological import and thus etiologically relevant. Rothman's theoretical framework of sufficient cause and component causes can be interpreted as a mechanistic model of causation, integrating both neurodevelopment and ongoing/prolonged neuro-inflammation processes that are intricately intertwined in autism etiology. Although this model does not per se provide new insights into autism etiology, it provides a framework for thinking about it. A similar conceptual model has previously been used in relation to cerebral palsy, described by its authors as a sequence of events leading to an outcome through causal chain or effect modification (Stanley, Blair, and Alberman 2000).

6.2.3.1 Sufficient causes, component causes

Let us reconsider the Mackie–Rothman model described in Section 2.4.1. In 1976, Ken Rothman defined a cause as "an act or event or a state of nature which initiates or permits, alone or in conjunction with other causes, a sequence of events resulting in an effect" (Rothman 1976). He suggested that disease occurrence always has multiple causes, and that "necessary" and "sufficient" causes should not be considered at the same explanatory level.

In Rothman's view, sufficient causes are causal constellations (often depicted as pies; see Figure 6.3) composed of units (pieces of a pie, each being called "component cause") that are either necessary (present in all sufficient causal constellations) or nonnecessary (present in some, but not all sufficient causal constellations). In essence, Rothman specifies three different categories of causes: (1) sufficient causes, represented by a whole pie; (2) necessary component causes, which are part (pieces) of all known possible sufficient causes (pies) of a disease of interest; and (3) nonnecessary component causes (pieces of some but not all pies), which are neither sufficient nor necessary. On this view of multifactorial causation, it is the unique combination and potentiation of necessary and nonnecessary component causes that will ultimately lead to illness occurrence. The obvious similarity to Mackie's concept of an insufficient but necessary part of an unnecessary but sufficient condition (Mackie 1965, 1974) is interesting but beyond the scope of this book.

In our mechanistic model, each pie represents one unique etiological pathway to autism, consisting of one unique combination of pathogenetic mechanisms that represent the perfect storm leading to autism. Each piece of each pie represents one pathogenetic mechanism, such as prematurity, neuro-inflammation, or genetics. Although components of pathogenetic mechanisms that give rise to each etiological pathway are not represented in Rothman's model, they could be displayed within each single piece of the pie. In essence, both etiological (pies) and pathogenetic

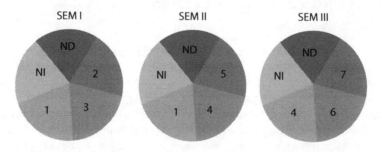

Figure 6.3 Model of sufficient etiological mechanisms (I, II, and III) composed of component causes that are either necessary (nPCMs, marked as ND and NI) or unnecessary (uPCMs, represented by numbers 1–7). (ND, neurodevelopment; NI, neuro-inflammation; SEM, sufficient etiological mechanism.)

mechanisms (pieces) can be conceived of as causal mechanisms at different (etiological versus pathogenetic) levels.

6.2.3.2 Etiological pathway as causal mechanism

In an article that suggests disease causation as the basis for disease classification systems, Severinsen states that

> if asked to give an objective answer to what the mechanism or the causal structure behind a disease is, one could argue that there are many "causal factors" in a complex structure of causes, and that, in most cases, those factors are neither sufficient nor necessary, but only contributory. (Severinsen 2001)

The use of the term *mechanism* in this passage coincides with a general surge of interest in mechanisms and mechanistic explanation in the philosophy of science over the past two decades. One frequently cited definition of *mechanism* is that of Machamer, Darden, and Craver: "Mechanisms are entities and activities organized such that they are productive of regular changes from start or set-up to finish or termination conditions" (2000:3).

In this sense of the term *mechanism*, the sufficient component cause model can integrate etiological and pathogenetic mechanisms of autism causation. Consider each sufficient cause (pie in Figure 6.3) representing a sufficient etiological mechanism (SEM). Each component cause (piece of the pie) represents one risk factor, one more basic fact we need to know about in order to understand the SEM. Moreover, each component cause (piece of pie) represents a pathogenetic component mechanism (PCM), either necessary (nPCM) or unnecessary (uPCM). In explanatory diagrams, candidate risk factors can be joined together inside one etiological pathway (SEM) by biologically plausible linkage points between elements of pathogenetic mechanisms in neighboring PCMs.

In keeping with this model, all identified risk factors of autism should be viewed primarily as candidate PCMs, which together form one SEM that is sufficient to create one version of the perfect storm leading to clinical autism. It is possible that different PCMs might make unequal contributions to our model. For example, as the incidence and severity of adverse neurodevelopmental outcomes increase with increasing degree of prematurity, the associated PCM might carry different weights depending on the gestational age at which a child was born. For a child born late or moderately preterm (32–36 weeks' gestation), the preterm birth-associated PCM might contribute to a lesser extent compared to that of a child born very preterm (28–31 weeks' gestation) or extremely preterm (less than 28 weeks' gestation). Since it is not known whether the risk for autism varies linearly with the degree of prematurity, further research is needed to better understand the contribution of various degrees of prematurity to our model.

Note that this model allows for multiple different etiological pathways to autism, each one represented by a different SEM. For example, up to about half of all autism cases appear to be attributable mainly to genetic factors (Gaugler et al. 2014; Iossifov et al. 2014). This means that genetics may be a uPCM (any piece of pie marked with a number 1–7 in Figure 6.3), because autism can occur without underlying genetic abnormalities, at least until good scientific evidence to the contrary becomes available. Prematurity is another uPCM, because autism can occur in children not born preterm. Similarly, male sex is a uPCM, as preterm boys are at higher risk for developing autism (Johnson et al. 2010).

This hypothetical framework could be explored through longitudinal studies involving biomarkers and examination of the neurometrics of functional imaging, in order to further enhance our understanding of autism causation and guide interventions for families of children at risk. Further research should also examine if this model is generalizable to all degrees of prematurity, to children with underlying genetic vulnerabilities, and to both sexes equally.

6.2.3.3 Interacting pathogenetic component mechanisms

In keeping with Carl Craver's suggestion to think of neuroscientific explanations as descriptions of multilevel mechanisms (Craver 2007), we suggest thinking of developmental neuroscientific explanations as descriptions of multilevel developmental mechanisms. Most developmentalists will agree that neurodevelopment is a neurobiological mechanism that eventually leads to the typical structure and function of the adult nervous system. Therefore, we argue that neurodevelopment is a causal process instantiated as one nPCM. While the process of neurodevelopment is still ongoing (beginning *in utero* and ending in early adulthood), a second nPCM (neuro-inflammation and/or ISSI) interacts with the first. In our explanatory model, microglia activation represents one pathogenetic mechanism within the nPCM neuro-inflammation, and neuronal migration toward the future cortex represents one pathogenetic mechanism within the nPCM neurodevelopment. The result is a deviation from the typical neurodevelopmental trajectory (the outcome at brain level) that is characterized by atypical function (the outcome at the clinical level).

6.2.4 Developmental causation

Rather than focusing on localized gene expression or environmental triggers as the main causal pathways to developmental disorders, Annette Karmiloff-Smith proposed thinking about these two essential pathogenetic mechanisms from a "neuroconstructivist" perspective (Karmiloff-Smith 1998). Her theory integrates the timing of gene expression and key interactions with other genetic and environmental factors, while taking into account the complex dynamics inherent to both normal and atypical human development. Rather than concentrating on a disorder or diagnosis when it significantly affects a child's functioning, Karmiloff-Smith suggests that it is of utmost importance to "study disorders in early infancy, and longitudinally, to understand how alternative developmental pathways might lead to different phenotypical outcomes."

The same developmental pathway might lead to different phenotypical outcomes at different time points during child development. Take, for example, the ongoing interaction between ISSI and neurodevelopmental mechanisms in the context of preterm brain damage (Malaeb and Dammann 2009; Volpe 2009). While damage to the developing brain structure will occur early, impairment of the developing function is not apparent until much later, when the demands of the environment exceed the capabilities of the child. Consequently, an early inflammatory insult "not only destroys what exists, but also changes what develops" (Malaeb and Dammann 2009). If we apply this theoretical framework to autism, it becomes clear that it is essential to study the atypical developmental processes early on, over time, and with consideration of multiple possible etiological scenarios (SEMs) for a specific clinical outcome. The proposed ongoing interaction between the neuro-inflammatory nPCM and the neurodevelopmental nPCM opens potential windows of opportunity at multiple times during childhood. Well-timed interventions could mechanistically target the ongoing pathogenetic processes during these windows of opportunity and modify the disease trajectory in a favorable direction.

6.3 PROCESS PERSPECTIVE IN ETIOLOGIC EXPLANATIONS

The main thrust of Section 6.2 is the proposal that autism is an ongoing *process*, not a static disorder. Thus, the distinction suggested is not between process and mechanism but between disease process and static disease. The argument is, basically, that it would be advantageous to study the etiology of autism from a developmental process perspective and not look at it as a disorder that suddenly pops up out of nowhere when some genetic or environmental cause happens to flick a biological or biopsychosocial switch. This perspective might be advantageous, because it would provide space for a discussion of candidate interventions at various stages of illness development. The classical genetic paradigm of autism holds that one of multiple known gene aberrations leads to the autistic phenotype and that we cannot do much about this. Taking the process perspective might offer multiple entry points for preventive or therapeutic intervention along the developmental pathway.

The paper that serves as the basis for Section 6.2 was my first attempt to take the etiological perspective by talking about causes, mechanisms, and processes in the natural history of autism. Based on my discussion in this book, some of the terms used previously should probably be clarified. This is done in Section 6.3.1. Thereafter, the mechanistic and process perspectives on etiological explanations are contrasted in Sections 6.3.2 and 6.3.3, respectively.

6.3.1 Terminological clarification

In Section 6.2, autism is referred to as an "etiologic process interfering with a second underlying process, that of typical neurodevelopment." Three points of clarification are in order.

First, reference was made to Rothman's sufficient-component cause model as a *mechanistic* model. In light of my discussion in this book, the model might better be viewed as integrating causes and pathomechanisms and, thus, be referred to as a causal-mechanical explanatory model.

Second, complete pies represented one etiological pathway to autism. If this pathway is the overarching *etiological process* as depicted in Figures 3.1 and 7.1, ranging from causes via pathomechanism to disease occurrence, each complete pie would depict a comprehensive etiological explanation.

Third, each piece of the pies was referred to as one pathogenetic mechanism. We should perhaps say instead that each piece of the pie can depict a cause *or* a pathomechanism. Thus, a whole pie would include the causal part, the pathomechanistic part, as well as other contributors discussed in Chapter 7.

In sum, the sufficient-component cause model can be interpreted as an etiological process model if (1) entire pies are taken to denote comprehensive etiological explanations that explain etiological processes, and (2) pieces of the pies are taken to represent causes or pathogenetic mechanisms that, taken together, make up the comprehensive etiological story we want to tell.

In the next two sections, previous explorations of what biomedical illness causation researchers mean when they talk about illness causation are expanded. Discussion zooms in on, and contrasts, two views of illness causation, as a *mechanism* and as a *process*. It is not my intention to *replace* the notion of mechanism with the notion of process. Rather, justification is provided of my suggestion to take a process perspective when building etiological explanations.

6.3.2 Mechanisms

Mechanisms have taken center stage in the philosophy of science.[5] As mentioned earlier, Machamer, Darden, and Craver's definition has mechanisms as "entities and activities organized such that they are productive of regular changes from start or set-up to finish or termination conditions" (2000).

Rothman's pies are conceptualized as SEMs that consist of constellations of component causes,[6] each of which can be seen as a PCM that can be either necessary (nPCM) or unnecessary (uPCM). Per my earlier clarification, the process perspective makes us see whole pies as sufficient etiological processes (SEPs) that consist of component causes and pathomechanisms. Together, these can form component causation processes (see Figures 3.1 and 7.1) that can be necessary or unnecessary.

Let's consider the following example of a comprehensive etiological explanation. Pediatric dermatologists Jenkins and coworkers explain the occurrence of tuberous sclerosis complex (TSC), a genetic multi-organ disease that affects the brain, skin, eye, and heart by way of abnormal tissue (i.e., tumor) generation, as follows:

> Tuberous sclerosis complex (TSC) is a disorder caused by mutations in the tumor suppressor genes TSC1 and TSC2, which encode the proteins hamartin and tuberin, respectively. This results in reduced inhibition of the mammalian target of rapamycin (mTOR) complex, which promotes cellular growth and proliferation. Clinically the disorder is characterized by development of benign hamartomatous neoplasms of various tissues. (Jenkins et al. 2016)

Here, the TSC1/TSC2 mutation is the purported *cause*, and reduced inhibition of growth promoter complex mTOR is the purported pathogenetic *mechanism* that explains *how* the genetic mutation causes the disease. The explanation also specifies two other component mechanisms (PCMs): first, abnormal hamartin and tuberin encoding, which links the cause (mutation) to the pathogenetic mechanism (lack of growth inhibition); and second, abnormal cell growth and proliferation, which links the pathogenetic mechanism to the disease (tuberous sclerosis). Thus, we have three mechanisms in between cause and clinical disease, and all together would qualify as a SEP that explains comprehensively *why* TSC comes about (gene mutation), and *how* (via abnormal hamartin and tuberin encoding, subsequent lack of growth inhibition, which leads to abnormal cell growth and proliferation).

None of these components alone is sufficient to lead to TSC because they are only components of the pie, which is sufficient iff (if and only if) it is complete. The question whether one of them (or both) is necessary or unnecessary is a question of whether there are SEPs other than the one that consists of the components listed that also explain the occurrence of tuberous sclerosis. This is the case because either one of the TSC1 and TSC2 gene mutations is capable of initiating lack of growth inhibition, the central pathomechanism that leads to TSC. Thus, neither TSC1 nor TSC2 is a necessary component cause of TSC.

Sometimes, however, authors attribute explanatory power only to the causes of illness, not the pathogenetic mechanism. Going back to the autism literature, one finds statements like this:

> A total of 134 healthcare workers participated in the study. In all, 78 (58.2%), 19 (14.2%) and 36 (26.9%) of the healthcare workers were of the opinion that the etiology of childhood autism can be explained by natural, preternatural and supernatural causes, respectively. (Bakare et al. 2009)

Or this one, again on autism spectrum disorders (ASDs):

> For the majority of individuals with ASD, the causes of the disorder remain unknown; however, in up to 25% of cases, a genetic cause can be identified. Chromosomal rearrangements as well as rare and *de novo* copy-number variants are present in ~10–20% of individuals with ASD, compared with 1–2% in the general population and/or unaffected siblings. Rare and *de novo* coding-sequence mutations affecting neuronal genes have also been identified in ~5–10% of individuals with ASD. (Huguet, Ey, and Bourgeron 2013)

Although the authors talk about causes in terms of the difference they make (mutations present in 10%–20% of ASD cases versus only 1%–2% in the general population), they do not talk about mechanisms. Others, however, do put mechanisms front and center in ASD etiology, in particular DNA methylation. Their argument is based on a syllogism:

> evidence demonstrate[es] that: (i) environmental factors contribute to determining individual ASD risk and/or severity; (ii) developmental exposures to environmental chemicals can alter DNA methylation in multiple tissues, including the brain; and changes in DNA methylation have been documented in autistic individuals and implicated in ASD pathogenesis. The question remaining is whether these events are causally linked. Currently, evidence pointing to changes in DNA methylation as a mechanism by which environmental chemicals contribute to ASD risk is limited [...] but the few studies that have addressed this question have potentially significant implications regarding the importance of environmental epigenetics in the etiology of ASD. (Keil and Lein 2016)

In essence, the authors infer that environmental chemicals are a cause for ASD via the mechanism of DNA methylation.[7]

Going back to TSC, Jenkins et al. are explicit about their mechanistic stance when they write "dysregulation of the mammalian target of rapamycin pathway is the underlying pathogenic mechanism in tuberous sclerosis complex" (Jenkins et al. 2016).[8] The apparent explanatory value of this decidedly mechanistic stance is further exemplified in the following quote from the abstract of another paper:

> Antiphospholipid antibody syndrome (APS) is an autoimmune acquired thrombophilia characterized by recurrent thrombosis and pregnancy morbidity in the presence of antiphospholipid antibodies (aPL). [...] The exact pathogenetic mechanism of APS is unknown, but different, not mutually exclusive, models have been proposed to explain how anti-PL autoantibodies might lead to thrombosis and pregnancy morbidity. (Negrini et al. 2016)

The keyword here is, of course, *pathogenetic mechanism*, which is deemed necessary to explain how the cause leads to the outcome. Nevertheless, one has to keep in mind that while some say that *mechanism* denotes the "causal structure behind a disease" (Negrini et al. 2016), it represents only that part of the "causal structure" that clarifies *how* disease occurs, not *why*.

Although the term *pathomechanism* is ubiquitous in biomedicine and biomedical research, some think that pathomechanisms do not even qualify as mechanisms in the first place. Justin Garson proposes a sense of mechanism that focuses on its *function*. His main claim is that "mechanisms serve functions [, which] places substantive constraints on the kinds of system activities 'for which' there can be a mechanism" (Garson 2013). Most interesting for my current discussion is that Garson further suggests that "there are no mechanisms for pathology. There is no mechanism for heart disease or Alzheimer's disease or schizophrenia because (e.g.,) heart disease on the part of a system is not a function of that system" (ibid.). Apparently, Garson uses the term *function* in a rather restrictive way to exclude *dys*function. The term *purpose* seems to fit his meaning well; he writes, for example, that "[t]he dolphin's fin can act as a hook that entangles the dolphin in nets. But it is not usually described as a mechanism for doing so. That is because getting entangled in nets is not its function" (p. 318).

Following are reasons for my disagreement. First, from the biomedical perspective, we do not (always) talk about mechanisms *for*. Instead, we talk about mechanisms *how*. We are interested in mechanisms and pathomechanisms precisely because we want to understand the mechanisms' function. We are not asking the teleological question *why* a mechanism does what it does, but the pragmatic one, *how* does it do it? Second, we are interested in the workings of biological mechanisms, which, at least for bioscientists, just *is* the mechanisms' function. In other words, biomedical function includes dysfunction, while Garsonian functionalists would need to exclude it. Consequently, they would not be able to construct comprehensive etiological explanations, unless they take the process perspective and talk about dysfunction as part of the etiological process.

6.3.3 Or process?

Etiology is the process of how illness comes about. Etiological explanations both require and generate knowledge about this process. Therefore, etiological explanations play a major role in medicine, epidemiology, the basic biomedical sciences, biomedical informatics, computational epidemiology, and medical malpractice litigation.[9] To review briefly, *causes* of illness are factors that induce and/ or affect illness occurrence; they are the beginning of the etiological pathway that leads from cause to effect, from initiator to illness. Most illness *causation* is biological, in the sense that causes and the remainder of the causation process (pathogenesis) constitute the etiologic explanation for illness occurrence. Taken as one process, the causes (e.g., ultraviolet radiation in skin cancer causation[10]) and the pathogenetic mechanism (e.g., failed repair of ultraviolet-radiation-induced cell damage[11]) form the basis for a comprehensive etiological explanation.

Another look at Machamer, Darden, and Craver's mechanisms ("entities and activities organized such that they are productive of regular changes from start or set-up to finish or termination conditions") makes it quite obvious that mechanisms can be conceived as *processes* (*from start or set-up to finish*) during which the production of regular changes happens. I suggest that the etiology of illness is described well as overlapping causation and disease processes, nested in the etiological process (Figures 3.1 and 7.1). Let us go over some *biological* notions of process.

In the biosciences, "mechanism" is often used synonymously with the dual notion that states that (1) there is a process (a *token* sequence of plausibly related phenomena) and (2) here is how it works (a *type* blueprint for sequences of the same kind).[12] Thus, can we think of all mechanisms in action as a process? Are some processes *not* mechanisms, that is, grief, a divorce, a safari? Waddington's epigenetic landscapes depict human development as a slanted surface of moguls with a ball rolling downhill in between them, and you never know where the ball might end up (Waddington 1957).

For some, the term *mechanism* has a rather deterministic connotation. For example, John Dupré suggests that

> There are good reasons to think that biological systems – organism, cells, pathways – are in many ways quite misleadingly thought of as mechanisms. (Dupré 2013:28)

Dupré's view is that mechanisms are machine-like.[13] This is what Nicholson has called the "*machine mechanism* sense of 'mechanism' (defined as) stable assemblies of interacting parts arranged in such a way that their combined operation results in predetermined outcomes" (Nicholson 2012:2). Dupré writes that it is not so much parts (=things) that "are stable and robust in biology, [...] but processes" (p. 30).

The term *process* is usually taken to mean "a sequence of events" (Blackburn 2016:385). William Bechtel writes that the idea of sequential ordering, which is equivalent to Rothman's "sequence of events resulting in an effect," makes it a "valuable first approach in explaining biological processes" (Bechtel 2011; emphasis mine). Thus, we can say that a description of the sequence of biological events (causes and mechanisms) that represents the *process of illness occurrence* qualifies as an etiological explanation.

According to the Gene Ontology Consortium, a biological process is defined as follows:

> A biological process is a recognized series of events or molecular functions. A process is a collection of molecular events with a defined beginning and end. Mutant phenotypes often reflect disruptions in biological processes.[14]

A biological process term describes a series of events accomplished by one or more organized assemblies of molecular functions. Examples of broad biological process terms are "cellular physiological process" or "signal transduction." Examples of more specific terms are "pyrimidine metabolic process" or "alpha-glucoside transport." The general rule to assist in distinguishing between a biological process and a molecular function is that a process must have more than one distinct step.

A biological process is not equivalent to a pathway. At present, the [gene ontology] does not try to represent the dynamics or dependencies that would be required to fully describe a pathway.[15]

The concept of constellations of multiple contributing causes, especially in a biomedical context, lends itself toward an interpretation from the causal process perspective, which holds that causation is to

be understood in terms of causal processes and interactions [and] any facts about causation as a relation between events obtain only on account of more basic facts about causal processes and interactions. (Dowe 2009)

Process views have a longstanding tradition in general philosophy (Rescher 1996, 2000; Whitehead 1929 [1960]) and in the philosophy of causation (Dowe 2000; Dowe 2009; Salmon 1984, 1998). What distinguishes a process from a mechanism? When Nicholson proposes that "in biology, the phenomenon produced by the causal *process* described in a causal mechanism usually enables the fulfillment of a function" (Nicholson 2012), the mechanism is considered a blueprint that describes the sequence of events (the process) that, in turn, produces a phenomenon that fulfills a function. Therefore, "specifying the causal mechanism for a function explains how this function is causally brought about" (ibid.).

One particularly interesting causal process theory (briefly discussed by Dowe) is Aronson's transference theory (Aronson 1971). Aronson discusses earlier work by Collingwood and Gasking, who proposed that all causal claims are ways of talking about related events in manipulationist, anthropomorphic ways and that any biological disease causation process that does not involve intelligent manipulation would, therefore, not be causal.[16] Thus, according to the Collingwood/Gasking view, none of the pathogenetic component causes of autism – the topic of Section 6.2 – can be considered a cause of autism. Aronson rejects the anthropomorphic view of causation and claims that "there are certain changes that take place in individuals that can be completely accounted for without having to appeal to the behavior of other individuals. I'll call these changes, 'natural changes'" (p. 421). He proposes an account of causation that conceptualizes any causal relationship between (cause) A and (effect) B to require (1) the change in B to be unnatural, (2) a physical contact between A and B at the time B occurs, and the transfer of a quantity from A to the object that displays the effect, manifesting as B. In essence, this proposal allows for any causation without human intervention, but it excludes all *developmental* changes in biology, because it "*contrasts* a caused change in a object with a change that would have taken place if it were left to itself" (ibid.; emphasis in original). Thus, according to Aronson, only nonnatural component causes of autism can be considered causes of autism. Since neurodevelopment is a natural process, it would not qualify as a cause of autism. Neither would any other biological cause qualify as such, which renders Aronson's theory useless for etiological explanations of ASD.

In my proposed etiological explanation of ASD, neurodevelopment qualifies as a cause via being a background condition. In a sense, neurodevelopment *contributes* to the etiology of ASD by virtue of being the biological process that causes, and pathomechanisms of ASD are piggybacking on so that, over time, the clinical ASD phenotype emerges.[17] In the next chapter, this framework is outlined and discussed further.

7 COMBINED CONTRIBUTION

7.1 INTRODUCTION

This chapter builds on previous sections by expanding on *causes versus conditions* (Section 4.4.3), *mechanism* (Chapters 5 and 6), and *process* (Chapter 6). My goal is to defend the position that background conditions such as socioeconomic status and other factors can *contribute* to the etiology of illness in ways that make a difference without being what is usually considered a cause. In essence, comprehensive etiological explanations may gain in explanatory depth if we include contributors whose role in the etiology of illness is not to initiate or induce the pathomechanism, but to interfere in other ways with the etiological process that make a difference to the outcome without fitting traditional definitions of a cause.

Section 7.2 is based on a previously published paper (Dammann 2017) written in response to a piece by Michael Kelly, Rachel Kelly, and Federica Russo (2014). The authors propose to integrate biological, behavioral, and social mechanisms into what they call *mixed mechanisms* that are situated in the individual's *lifeworld*. In response, terminological discrepancies were discussed, and their pathogenetic perspective was replaced with my *etiological stance*, which includes, but is not limited to, pathogenesis (Figure 7.1). Also discussed was whether the lifeworld concept adds to what we consider an individual's environment. It was also suggested, and this brings me to the topic of this chapter, that the notion of *mixed mechanisms* be replaced with the concept of *combined contributions* in etiological explanations of illness.

In Section 7.3, more detail is added to what was written in the original paper by showing how etiological explanations could become more comprehensive and perhaps even more useful when enhanced by the notion of combined contribution. For starters, a model that includes inducers, modifiers, and mediators as potential contributors to etiological processes is outlined (Figure 7.2).

7.2 EXPLAINING ILLNESS OCCURRENCE

Models of illness causation play a crucial role in medicine and public health. In their recent paper on this topic, Michael Kelly, Rachel Kelly, and Federica Russo state that the integration of social, biological, and behavioral causes in the same etiological mechanism remains to be clarified. In particular, they think that current models of illness causation do not appreciate "the truly integrated nature of bio-social-behavioral

ETIOLOGY

... the story that explains illness occurrence

Causes ➔ Pathogenesis
(Pathogenetic mechanism) ➔ Clinical
disease

⬌ Causation process

⬌ Disease process

⬌ Etiological process

Figure 7.1 The *etiological stance* conceptualizes etiology as a two-step process. The first phase (*causation process*) includes causes and the subsequent pathogenetic mechanisms they induce. The second phase (*disease process*) includes the pathogenesis and clinical disease. Knowledge about both (*etiological process*), combined with knowledge about the actions of other contributors to the etiological process at all levels, can provide useful etiological explanations.

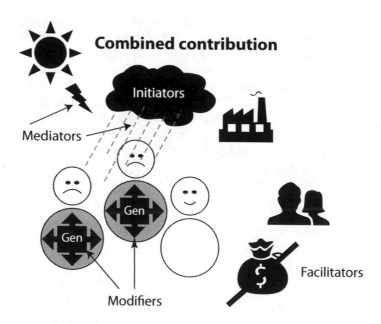

Figure 7.2 *Combined contribution* is the view that talk about causes is less useful than talk about the joint role of all etiological factors that contribute to illness occurrence. Such factors are, for example, causal initiators/inducers of pathogenesis (depicted as sun and toxic cloud), causal mediators (radiation and rain), genetic susceptibility modifiers, and social facilitators (e.g., gender bias, poverty), among many other possibilities.

pathogenesis" (Kelly, Kelly, and Russo 2014:309). In brief, they suggest that (1) two levels of explanation are at work in medicine and public health – biological and social; (2) integration is difficult because of resistance to including social determinants of disease in both the biomedical and social sciences; and (3) we should "move to an integrated model, where biological and social factors are ontologically equivalent, in the sense that both have a role in disease etiology" (p. 310).

The authors begin to support their argument by describing what they call "the original public health vision" of medical and public health pioneers, including Snow, Virchow, and Duncan, who "did not demonstrate empirically what today would be defined as the biological causes of disease, [but] they gathered enough circumstantial evidence to show the associations between poor social conditions and disease, and they intervened on the basis of that circumstantial evidence" (p. 312). Kelly, Kelly, and Russo (KKR) think that recent developments in public health have led to "the separation of the social from the biological and of the individual from the population" (p. 311). They proceed by outlining current views of social causation: George Engel's biopsychosocial model, the Sussers' eco-epidemiology, Geoffrey Rose's causes of causes, and Nancy Krieger's web of causation (Engel 1977; Krieger 1994; Rose 1992; Susser 2004), But, alas, all accounts fall short of their expectations, because even their favorite one (Krieger's) does not "stress fully enough the explanatory import of social factors or the social level of explanation and their connection with the biological" (p. 316).

In order to fill that void, KKR suggest using social categories not just as descriptive characteristics of individuals and populations, which, they hold, masks "the active causal role of social factors in the etiology of diseases" (p. 317). Instead, they propose that "Social categories should not be mere classificatory devices, but *explanatory devices*" (ibid.; emphasis in original). They use the term *lifeworld* to mean the sum of all social and material factors that are relevant to humans in their immediate environment. In this sense, they argue, an individual's lifeworld includes the "physical, economic, social, and microbiological" causes of disease (ibid.).

The authors also suggest that the establishment of causal claims in the health sciences requires evidence of both statistical correlation and pathogenetic mechanism. This claim, the topic of Chapter 5 in this book, holds that we need evidence of not only correlation[1] between candidate causes (risk factors) and health outcomes but also mechanisms linking the two (Russo and Williamson 2007b). In this context, evidence of association, sometimes referred to by philosophers as evidence of difference-making, is evidence of a statistical association between risk factors and diseases. It has been suggested that this kind of evidence should be called "exposure-outcome evidence," at least in epidemiological contexts.[2] Evidence of mechanism, on the other hand, is evidence of biological processes that involve chemical reactions or other kinds of biological signal transduction. While KKR appear to accept that associations between social and biological factors are appreciated in biomedicine, they hold that full acceptance as causes of illness would require the demonstration of *how* they are connected mechanistically. As one possible realization of what they call "mixed mechanisms" of disease development, they discuss epigenetics, the phenomenon of noninherited, environmental-induced changes to genetic information.

My goal in this chapter is to show that what is convincing in KKR's argument (integrate social and biological factors) is not new, and what is new (mixed mechanisms) is not convincing. First, a few thoughts are offered about the dichotomy of original versus current visions of public health (as perceived by Kelly, Kelly, and Russo). Clarification is provided on how the terms *process* and *mechanism* are used in this chapter. Second, four brief suggestions are given on how to modify and build on the thesis by KKR.

7.2.1 Original versus current visions of public health

Kelly, Kelly, and Russo claim that classic pioneers of public health did not demonstrate mechanisms, such as John Snow (1813–1858), who discovered the association between certain sources of drinking water and cholera incidence during an outbreak in London in 1854.[3] But how could they without access to the concepts and machinery needed to do proper molecular microbiology? Moreover, we still rely on circumstantial evidence in some of our most successful public health interventions in the twentieth and twenty-first centuries. For example, smoking cessation clearly reduces mortality, although the mechanism by which smoking causes deadly lung disease is still incompletely understood today (Anthonisen et al. 2005; Cooper et al. 2013). Knowledge of pathogenetic mechanisms is not needed for public health intervention, although it is obviously crucial for the development of pharmacomedical interventions that target such mechanisms (more on this later in this chapter). Most importantly, however, current public health still promotes the idea that biological and social factors play equally important roles in models of disease causation. In his proposal to move from risk factors to explanations in public health, Ian McDowell asked for explanations that

> should span several layers of causal processes. They should incorporate a plausible theory, or theories, that trace the connections between the levels. There should be an analysis both of the dynamics of the process ("why did this occur?"); and of its functioning ("how do the processes operate?"). (McDowell 2008:223)

Of note, McDowell uses the term *causal process*, not m*echanism*. Perhaps those of us who work in public health and epidemiology are a bit more process oriented and less mechanistically inclined than basic biomedical researchers. Indeed, I had a similar scenario in mind when writing that

> systems epidemiology adds yet another level consisting of antecedents that might contribute to the disease process in populations. In etiologic and prevention research, systems-type thinking about multiple levels of causation will allow epidemiologists to identify contributors to disease at multiple levels as well as their interactions. (Dammann et al. 2014)

Let's briefly summarize again the differences between *process* and *mechanism* as the terms are used in this book. First, both are used in the context of the story that explains illness occurrence, the *etiology* of illness. In the epidemiological tradition, etiology is defined as a three-step process (Figure 7.1), beginning with initiating causal events and subsequent mechanisms in the body that culminate in clinically visible disease, which may or may not undergo phenotype changes over time, often referred to as its "clinical course" (MacMahon and Pugh 1970). Thus defined, the etiological process includes causes, pathogenesis, and disease. The etiological process can be subdivided into the illness causation process, including causes and pathogenesis, which overlaps with the disease process, which includes pathogenesis and the clinical course of disease. Pathogenesis (etiology minus initial causes and subsequent disease) is often considered a *mechanism* and sometimes called *pathomechanism*.

These epidemiological views are in keeping with philosophical definitions. For example, the *Oxford Dictionary of Philosophy* has this for the *process* entry: "a sequence of events" (Blackburn 2016). The definition of *mechanism*, in its probably most frequently cited version in recent philosophy of science, is a bit more complicated: "(m)echanisms are entities and activities organized such that they are productive of regular changes from start or set-up to finish or termination conditions" (Machamer, Darden, and Craver 2000:3). In biology, dynamic explanations often describe phenomena that are not sequential but include complex cyclic feedback loops (Bechtel 2011). Thus, this author endorses what Bechtel calls "dynamic mechanistic explanations" when it comes to biological explanations of pathogenetic phenomena. His definition for this kind of mechanism is

> a structure performing a function in virtue of its component parts, component operations, and their organization. The orchestrated functioning of the mechanism, manifested in patterns of change over time in properties of its parts and operations, is responsible for one or more phenomena. (Bechtel and Abrahamsen 2010:323)

Using these definitions for *process* and *mechanism*, the natural history of illness occurrence can be seen as proceeding sequentially from causes via pathomechanisms to illness. In this etiological process, the pathomechanism of a certain disease is the internal dynamic biological mechanism that explains the apparent link between external causes and clinical illness.

Now we go back to public health. In what is called the "expanded host-agent-environment paradigm," biological as well as social factors are considered characteristics of both the host and the environment. The environment can be involved in this process in at least two ways: first, by contributing "factors to host susceptibility; for example, unemployment, poverty, or low education level" (Tulchinsky and Varavikova 2009:49); and second, by contributing the agents that induce the disease process – in other words, infectious or noninfectious factors mainly of biological nature. Much of this multilevel illness causation model has been developed and is being cogently promoted by Galea and colleagues:

> First, factors at multiple levels, including biological, behavioural, group and macro-social levels, all have implications for the production and distribution of health. Secondly, these factors frequently influence one another and, in addition, are sometimes influenced by the health indicators of interest. (Galea, Riddle, and Kaplan 2010:98)

Moreover, mechanisms of how social factors are biologically linked to health outcomes have been documented in the basic science literature for quite some time. For example, Eisenberger and Cole have summarized evidence in support of the claim that "social connections reach deep into the body to regulate some of our most fundamentally internal molecular processes," and they predict that "social neuroscience approaches will be important for deciphering both how and why social relationships are critical for health" (Eisenberger and Cole 2012:673).

In other words, contrary to KKR's conception, the current public health paradigm of illness causation *does* integrate biological and social factors and considers them equally important; however, both play multiple roles as characteristics of both the individual and his or her environment – or what KKR call *lifeworld* – and can function as modifiers of susceptibility and as inducers of pathogenetic mechanisms.

7.2.2 Terminology matters

Two points should be mentioned with regard to KKR's usage of disease causation terminology. First, they use the terms *etiology* and *pathogenesis* as if they are interchangeable. They are not. As previously outlined, *etiology* is the entire process that leads to illness occurrence, while *pathogenesis* is the intrapersonal pathophysiological mechanism that explains the link between causes and clinical illness (Figure 7.1). On this view, pathogenesis is both the intra-individual second stage of the disease causation process and also the first stage of the disease process.

Second, I disagree with KKR's interpretation of the common usage of *proximal* and *distal* causes of disease as synonymous with *biological* and *social*. The original proposal to distinguish two kinds of causes in biology goes back to Ernst Mayr (1904–2005), who wrote in 1961 that "proximate causes govern the responses of the individual (and his organs) to immediate factors of the environment while ultimate causes are responsible for the evolution of the particular DNA code" (Mayr 1961:1503). In contrast to both KKR, and Mayr, and in keeping with my distinction between processes and mechanisms in disease etiology, refer to elements of pathogenetic, micro-etiological mechanisms as *proximal*, and to pre-pathogenetic, macro-etiological risk factors (candidate causes) that induce, facilitate, or modify pathogenetic mechanisms, as *distal*. While pathogenetic mechanisms are mainly, and perhaps exclusively, biochemical functional networks, macro-etiological factors can be biological (such as microbes), physical (ambient particulate matter), or social (poverty). In this sense, distal causes and proximal mechanisms are also indicators of the time sequence of the illness development process, to wit the etiology of illness.

7.2.3 Etiological stance

Regarding KKR's request to use social characteristics as explanatory devices, social epidemiologists will respond that this is in fact exactly what they do already. Mervyn Susser (1921–2014), a champion of social epidemiology and prominent advocate for rigorous causal thinking in his discipline, wrote that "epidemiology is the study of the distribution and determinants of states of health in human populations," and that "a determinant can be any factor … so long as it brings about change for better or worse in a health condition" (Susser 1973:3). Accordingly, today's social epidemiologists define their trade as "the branch of epidemiology that studies the social distribution and social determinants of states of health" (Berkman and Kawachi 2000:6). Both

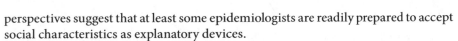

perspectives suggest that at least some epidemiologists are readily prepared to accept social characteristics as explanatory devices.

Illness causation is better captured in an etiological framework, not just a pathogenetic one. Following MacMahon and Pugh (1970:26), the term *etiological stance* is used to refer to the *causal process* that includes causal induction and pathogenetic mechanism, which overlaps with the *disease process,* which includes pathogenetic mechanism and clinical disease. The former spans the time from first exposure to a risk factor to the end of the pathogenetic mechanism. The latter begins with the pathogenetic mechanism and includes all of the clinical course of the disease of interest.

Note that factors that play a role during the causation process (e.g., inducers, modifiers, mediators) are viewed as *any* kind of state (such as socioeconomic status), event (exposure to asbestos), or behavior (eating vegetables) that can be thought of as playing a biologically plausible role in determining the beginning of a pathogenetic mechanism. In this conceptual framework, etiological knowledge comprises knowledge about the entire process, including knowledge about pre-pathogenetic causes (generated mainly by epidemiologists) and knowledge about pathogenetic mechanisms (generated mainly by bench scientists). Again, knowledge about pathogenetic mechanisms is needed mainly for the development of pharmacomedical interventions, while knowledge about causes is often sufficient for disease prevention.

7.2.4 Bio-social lifeworlds

Kelly, Kelly, and Russo use the term *lifeworld* to describe the space in which human relationships, as well as other social, biological, and physical environmental characteristics, function as portals for adverse exposures. Rudolf Virchow (1821–1902) used the term "living conditions" (*Lebensbedingungen*) when describing his view of the primacy of external causes in the form of changes in altered living conditions on heritable acquired characteristics (*"eine erbliche Variation irgend einmal durch eine Causa externa, durch eine Veränderung der Lebensbedingungen entstanden sein muss"*) (Wenig 1998–99:221).

The usage of the term *lifeworld* by Kay S. Toombs in her discussion of George Engel's biopsychosocial account of the physician's and patient's lifeworlds (Toombs 1992) suggests that KKR's vision of mixed mechanisms is identical, or at least compatible with, the disease model of psychosomatic medicine, which has been called "the scientific foundation of the biopsychosocial model" (Novack et al. 2007). It is the standard view of psychosomatic medicine that social factors play an enormous role as health determinants, not only as initiators of the disease process, but also as protectors in the form of social support (Cobb 1976). Thus, one is left wondering what KKR's proposal offers beyond the biopsychosocial and psychosomatic models of illness causation.

7.2.5 Combined contribution

Kelly, Kelly, and Russo propose "mixed mechanisms" as a concept to bring social and biological mechanisms together in the individual's lifeworld. I think that what they envision might be better described as "combined contribution" (Figure 7.2).

7.2.5.1 Mechanism

Although Kelly, Kelly, and Russo think that an integrated model of disease causation should allow social and biological factors to interact mechanistically, they do not explain how this overarching mechanism could look (form) and work (function). They use the lifeworld image to circumscribe the space where they see such a mechanism taking place, and they use epigenetics as an example of a current research field in which "mixed mechanisms are at work."

Kelly, Kelly, and Russo describe *epigenetics* as a link between social and biological mechanisms in disease causation. This is an interesting example but too narrow a view of existing models of sociobiological causation. A full-fledged discussion of epigenetics would go far beyond the scope of this chapter. Briefly, noninherited environmentally induced changes in the genetic makeup (specifically in DNA methylation status) of individuals can provide a link between environmental factors and biological responses. As causally suggestive titles of scientific reports on epigenetic findings may be – such as "Social crowding during development causes changes in GnRH1 DNA methylation" (Alvarado et al. 2015) – I do not see how such a mechanism is *mechanistically* different from others that link social causes and biological pathogenetic mechanisms. For example, social considerations appear to be the major driver among adolescents for their risky tanning behavior, which increases their exposure to ultraviolet radiation, whose cutaneous carcinogenicity is mechanistically well understood (Pfeifer and Besaratinia 2012; Sjoberg et al. 2004).

Although the epigenetics example is an interesting one, it does not offer an explanation of how social forces in a person's lifeworld result in epigenetic events at the genetic level. The authors suggest that "studying these epigenetic marks may provide the previously unknown mechanistic links between genetics, disease, and the environment" (Kelly, Kelly, and Russo 2014:320). Nowhere do they even allude to the idea that the form and function of at least some integrated sociobiological mechanisms are actually known.

Reverse mechanisms, to wit explanations of how biological factors determine social behaviors, have been studied by E. O. Wilson (1980). Although such mechanisms might be equally important in the context of illness causation, KKR do not refer to these at all, probably because they lament the perceived lack of attention to mechanisms that integrate socio-causal explanations with existing biological ones, not the lack of attention to mechanisms that integrate bio-causal explanations with accepted social ones. Still, if their idea is to integrate both in one model, both directions are worthy of consideration as components of a comprehensive account of etiology of illness.

However, why is it necessary to bring up mechanisms at all? The past decades have brought forward a great number of publications in the philosophy of science literature that define and discuss mechanisms and causality in the context of science and of biology, medicine, and epidemiology (Bechtel 2008, 2011; Bechtel and Abrahamsen 2005; Bechtel and Richardson 1993; Broadbent 2011; Clarke et al. 2013b; Craver and Darden 2013; Erdei and Dammann 2014; Garson 2013; Glennan 1996; Illari and Williamson 2012; Kincaid 2011; Machamer, Darden, and Craver 2000; Nicholson 2012; Williamson 2011a,b). As explained earlier and as depicted in Figure 7.1, the term *process* is used here to describe the entire etiological story of disease occurrence, close to or perhaps even synonymous to Lewis's "causal history" (Lewis 1986). Although the term *mechanism* (in Bechtel's sense of dynamic mechanism) is used, the preference is to abstain from the term altogether, mainly because the term does not fit biological phenomena well. First, it is, in general, unclear as to what a mechanism is, as indicated by the multiple available definitions (Illari and Williamson 2012). Second, unless tweaked to include cyclic organization of phenomena, the term appears to be too rigid to capture the fact that biological signaling networks are quite stable and robust over generations despite their flexibility to adapt (Bechtel 2011). Third, definitions of *mechanism* include too broad a range of reference to things and functions, for example, "entities" and "activities" (Machamer, Darden, and Craver 2000), "interactions between parts" (Glennan 2002), and "parts" and "operations" (Bechtel and Abrahamsen 2005). Fourth, this raises the possibility that "there is a serious danger of vacuity ... that mechanisms just are whatever explains whatever happens" (Dupré 2013). One suggestion in response to at least two of these considerations is to replace *mechanism* with *process* in etiological explanations, because what is "stable and robust in biology are not things, but processes" (Dupré 2013). A full-fledged defense of this proposal has to wait for another time.

7.2.5.2 Explanation

Kelly, Kelly, and Russo subscribe to the Russo–Williamson thesis (RWT), the view that to "establish causal relations we typically need both evidence of correlation and evidence of mechanisms" (Kelly, Kelly, and Russo 2014:316). Alex Broadbent, conversely, has observed that the history of epidemiology suggests that intervention on causal claims without mechanistic evidence can be very successful, as in the examples of John Snow and cholera, and Ignaz Semmelweis (1818–1865) and childhood fever. He concludes that his vignettes "cast doubt on the usefulness of a methodological principle stating that discovery of mechanisms is necessary for warranted causal inference" (Broadbent 2011:57). However, in order to offer comprehensive etiological explanations, knowledge about the entire etiological process is needed, including both causal and pathogenetic components.

Here the question arises, what exactly do we do when we explain? One answer is that to give a causal explanation for "an event is to provide some information about its causal history" (Lewis 1986:217). Although such causal history can already be interpreted as being equivalent to what we mean by *etiology* (including both causal and pathogenetic components), Salmon's "causal/mechanical explanation" fits the bill even better. He actually used the term *etiological explanation* – borrowing it from Wright (1976) – to refer to "a causal network consisting of relevant causal interactions that occurred previously and suitable causal processes that connect them to the fact-to-be-explained" (Salmon 1984:269). Salmon also referred to kinds of explanation that place emphasis on "the causal behavior of the constituents ... rather than upon a set of antecedent causes" (p. 270). He called this kind of explanation "constitutive explanation," which seems equivalent to what is now called *mechanistic explanation*. Lewis's "causal history" is potentially synonymous with the epidemiological meaning of *etiology*, although his definition of "causal explanation" is silent about mechanisms that connect causes and effects. Salmon and Wright's "etiological explanation," however, is clearly an explanation of a disease's etiology as used here, because it includes information about both the antecedent causes and suitable pathogenetic mechanisms.

7.2.5.3 Contribution

One has to be mindful of the close link between knowledge and action, in medicine and in public health. All action in medicine and public health needs to be justified, and knowledge based on evidence is the Big Justifier. What kind of evidence do we need to generate knowledge that is solid enough to justify action? Instead of relying solely on causal claims, based on separate evidence of difference-making and evidence of mechanism (Russo and Williamson 2007b), we may want to consider relying on evidence of contribution, which can come as either evidence of difference-making or of mechanism, or both.

Viewed from the pragmatic angle, it might be most helpful to spike etiological explanations with knowledge about all kinds of contributors to illness occurrence, including, but not limited to, causal initiators/inducers of pathogenesis (depicted as sun and toxic cloud in Figure 7.2), causal mediators (radiation and rain), genetic susceptibility modifiers, and social facilitators (e.g., gender bias, poverty), among many other possibilities My suggestion to move from causation to *combined contribution* echoes Morten Severinsen, who wrote that

> One of the problems which the principle of objective disease mechanism gives rise to, is that diseases are multifactorially conditioned (e.g., by having a so-called multifactorial etiology): If asked to give an objective answer to what the mechanism or the causal structure behind a disease is, one could argue that there are many "causal factors" in a complex structure of causes, and that, in most cases, those factors are neither sufficient nor necessary, but only contributory. (Severinsen 2001:322)

For example, one epidemiological scenario in which one factor contributes to the causal process by modifying the link between a certain exposure and a certain disease is *effect modification*. Effect modification occurs in any situation in which individuals in two (or more) subgroups, defined by a variable called the *effect modifier*, differ quantitatively with regard to the respective exposure-outcome association. Such effect modification "is a finding to be reported rather than a bias to be avoided" (Rothman and Greenland 1998:254). Effect modification is one method in which epidemiologists honor the proposal by KKR to invoke both biological and social explanations for their findings. Consider the following quotation from the abstract of a real-life epidemiological study:

> Job related mechanical exposure in both sexes, and psychosocial factors in women, seem independently of each other to play a part for development of shoulder and neck pain in vocationally active people. The effect of psychosocial factors was more prominent in women, which could be the result of biological factors as well as gender issues. These results suggest that interventions aiming at reducing the occurrence of shoulder and neck pain should include both mechanical and psychosocial factors. (Ostergren et al. 2005)

The upshot of this conclusion is that biological, psychosocial, and mechanical factors can be readily identified and put together in an integrated explanation of their combined contributions to shoulder and knee pain, which can be used as a step toward helpful interventions. However, despite the recognition of multifactorial disease models in the medical and lay communities, current etiological research is still dominated by attempts to identify "independent risk factors," presumably causal antecedents of illness that contribute to illness occurrence independent of others. The underlying idea appears to be that by identifying "independent risk factors," one identifies necessary causes of illness, which would reduce illness occurrence if avoided. However, the tension between attempts to identify (in practice) independent preventable risk-reducing factors and the acknowledgment (in theory) that there is no such thing as a single cause of illness deserves consideration. The current "conception of multifactorial causes" holds that

> all kinds of causal factors form a "causal complex," "causal web" or "web of causation" that contributes to the development of a disease. Each factor is neither necessary nor sufficient, for producing the disease state, but their combination and potentiation lead to the effect. (Dekkers and Rikkert 2006)

Replacement of notions of causation with notions of contribution would require more than a mere change in terminology. In particular, I think that the overly simplistic folk concept of illness causation ("one cause, one disease") prevents some etiological factors that are not direct inducers of illness from being considered in etiological explanations. Any factor that facilitates illness onset, changes susceptibility, or modifies illness risk contributes to illness occurrence. Therefore, we should assemble all of these factors, together with direct causes, under the term *contributor* and denote their collective action as "combined contribution."

Replacing narrow notions of causation with wider notions of contribution at all etiological levels will hopefully redirect attention away from single causes and toward a more holistic explanation of etiological processes. Kelly, Kelly, and Russo's contribution is a very important step in the right direction, one that can perhaps be improved along the lines discussed. To comprehensively explain complex etiologies, we need comprehensive, flexible concepts. In what follows, this proposal is outlined in more detail.

7.3 CONTRIBUTORS TO ILLNESS OCCURRENCE

Some, and perhaps even most, etiological explanations are qualitatively different from other examples of causal-mechanical explanations, such as why and how flipping a light switch makes a difference by making the room seem lighter or darker. Etiological explanations of some diseases have become so complex that the disease is actually called a "complex disease."[4] Over the centuries, health scientists have developed techniques that help them generate more comprehensive etiological explanations. What makes etiological explanations more comprehensive is when more details can be added to the story of how disease develops.

In the remainder of this chapter, some examples are offered of *what kind of* factors would qualify. In brief, any factor, broadly conceived as a sociological, psychological,

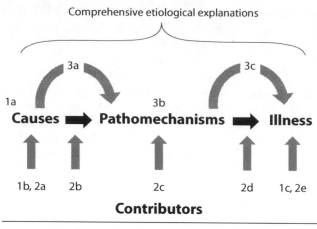

Figure 7.3 Inducers, modifiers, and mediators are contributors to etiological processes.

or physico-biological fact or event, that makes a measurable contribution to illness occurrence should qualify. The term *contributor* is used because it includes all factors that contribute to outcome occurrence (Figure 7.3), including factors that induce, modify, mediate, or moderate the etiological process at the level of the cause, the pathogenesis, or the illness.

7.3.1 Kinds of contribution

A framework for etiological explanations that replaces talk about causes with talk about contributors, without suggesting to replace causes with contributors, was suggested. Instead, look at causes as only one of multiple classes of factors that contribute to the etiology of illness. On this view, all causes are contributors, but not all contributors are causes (Figure 7.2). In epidemiology, causes are usually those factors or events that *initiate* the etiological process. But there are other kinds of contributors and conditions that are not usually considered to be causes. Here, the term *cause* is used in this epidemiological sense, not in the (many) broader senses that populate the philosophical literature.

Here is a first attempt to define *etiological contributors (ECs)*.

EC: A contributor to a health outcome is any factor that is part of and plays a functional role in an etiological process.

So defined, meddling with a contributor will likely change outcome occurrence; it will make a difference. However, we are not (yet) prepared to make difference-making a criterion for all kinds of contribution. Still, some sort of manipulationist framework of contribution might be helpful, simply because the goal of medicine and public health is to intervene in order to reduce the burden of illness. Thus, it seems prudent to include only contributors that, when changed, yield changes in health outcomes. However, this would be a mistake. We should not exclude contributors that cannot be modified for the purpose of health improvement, such as age or race. If such factors make a difference in outcome, they will still enrich our etiological explanations. And even if they do not make a measurable difference in outcome, they still make a contribution to such difference-making. One example would be redundancies, as they often occur in biology. If a pathomechanism such as inflammation works via receptor activation of one pro-inflammatory cytokine, a similar receptor for a related cytokine might be a passive bystander until the reservoir of the first cytokine is exhausted. The bystander would then become an active part of the pathomechanism. I think that the second cytokine-receptor pair should count as a contributor to the pathomechanism if only in its bystander function as a backup.

Some process theories of causation (in particular Salmon's) employ the criterion of *mark transmission*. The idea is Reichenbach's, who used the term *mark* the way we now use the term *difference*, as in difference-making (Reichenbach 1957:136).[5] Reichenbach writes that his "definition of causal connection considers the causal chain a signal, that is, the transmission of a mark" (p. 271). Salmon initially adopted this criterion for his distinction between causal processes from pseudo-processes (Salmon 1984:142) and later agreed with Dowe's suggestion to replace the mark transmission criterion with one of conserved quantities (Dowe 1995; Salmon 1997). It is not my goal to review this discussion here, but mark transmission as in *sending a signal* would be a good description for what is going on in etiological processes.

At the etiological level, a cause is that first step in the causation process that initiates the pathomechanism, and the pathomechanism is the biological mechanism that initiates the disease process (Figures 7.1 and 7.2). Here, the cause sends a signal that initiates the pathomechanisms, which in turn culminates in a signal that leads to clinical illness. The term *contributor* is used here for all entities that are involved in the sending (causes), changing (modifying), or transduction (mediation) of signals in the etiological process, be it biological, psychological, or social signals. One objection is that, at a certain level way down in the biological swamp of molecules, peptides, and their receptors, *all* of these contributors are causes, because whatever they do to help drive the etiological process forward, they must do it by causing a change. My response is that all components of complex etiological processes can be viewed as playing different roles when viewed from different angles. From this perspectivist vantage point, etiological explanations and their components can differ depending on the observer's interest, just as all explanations are interest-relative in one way or another.

We want to be as inclusive as possible for a very pragmatic reason. We cannot afford, in medicine or public health, to miss any potentially actionable target for intervention that would help reduce the burden of illness. Even if some components of the etiological process cannot be acted on directly, they still may increase our knowledge of what is going on in an etiological process, which may help identify *other* actionable target entities. Therefore, we should consider all kinds of factors involved in the etiological process, including, for example, inducers (senders of signals), modifiers (changers of signals), and mediators (carriers of signals), all of which come in various social and biological shapes and colors.

The idea of a contributor is not mine, and it is not new. This idea is being discussed as reflected in the Mackie–Rothman INUS-Pie model of sufficient and component causes (in Section 2.4.1). Mackie developed his notion INUS based on J. S. Mill's admittedly rather determinist statement that "[i]t is usually between the consequent and the sum of several antecedents; the concurrence of all of them being requisite to produce, that is, to be certain of being followed by, the consequent."[6] This concurrence of multiple contributors to the causal process is also reflected in David Lewis's suggestion that explaining a particular event is to tell its "long and complicated causal history. We might imagine a world where causal histories are short and simple; but in the world as we know it, the only question is whether they are infinite or merely enormous" (Lewis 1986:214). Modern bioscientists build on this assumption and try to tell the etiological story by drawing on different kinds of evidence and different interacting kinds of causal contribution. While the Lewis quote refers to particular (token) events, he also spoke to the issue of kinds of (type) events:

> information may be provided about what is common to all the parallel causal histories – call it *general explanatory information* about events of the given kind. To explain a kind of event is to provide some general explanatory information about events of that kind. (Lewis 1986:225; italics is cursive in original)

This is exactly what epidemiologists do: identify kinds of etiological explanations by providing general explanatory information that consists of plausible and true data about what is common to their causal histories.

In Section 7.2, I wrote about KKR's article that "what is new isn't convincing and what is convincing isn't new" is written about. The same could be said about my proposal if the two main notions of our respective proposals (mixed mechanisms versus combined contribution) were semantically equivalent. They are not. KKR subscribe to the view put forward by the RWT, that "to establish causal relations we typically need both evidence of correlation and evidence of mechanisms" (Kelly, Kelly, and Russo 2014:316). Looking through the epidemiological lens, we first talk about causes of illness in a more restricted way, referring only to the inducers of etiological processes (Figure 7.1). Second, we take the illness *causation process* to be the sum of the causes and the pathomechanisms they induce, and the *disease process* to be the sum of the pathomechanisms and the clinical disease (yes, they overlap by both including the pathogenetic mechanism). One could say that the KKR/RWT way to explain illness occurrence (what they call "explain disease") (Kelly, Kelly, and Russo 2014:316) is a shift toward inclusion of contributors that are not direct producers of their effects and will broaden the field of discussion.

We would benefit from a more flexible concept of etiological thinking and causal inference that does exactly what doctors and researchers might often *not* be interested in, namely, provide descriptions of the entire "causal complex" or "causal connection" of diseases with a multivariable etiological story (Dekkers and Rikkert 2006). However, such flexible etio-theory needs to offer room for "fuzzy" techniques of data analysis and causal inference, and probably most importantly, must let go of notions of "true causes of disease."[7] Fourth, enhancing notions of causation with notions of contribution might redirect the attention of researchers, physicians, nurses, and other healthcare workers from single elusive bits toward an understanding (or its absence) of etiologic wholes by appreciating comprehensive etiological explanations.

In what follows is described how certain parts of those causal histories provide different kinds of general explanatory information. The concept of contribution is described in detail by giving examples for three different kinds of contributors, that is, inducers, mediators, and moderators. Of course, this is not an exhaustive list and can probably be expanded appreciably in interesting ways.

7.3.2 Induction

The importance given to the term *exposure* by epidemiologists reflects the assumption that it is the first of multiple events that lead to illness and, thus, *induces* the etiological process (in the sense of initiating it). In traditional and molecular epidemiology, such inducers are often called the "exposure of interest" (Schulte and Perera 1993:6). Inducers are often considered "the cause" of the etiological process (item #1a in Figure 7.3). They start the etiological process, and the exposure of an individual to an inducer is thought of as the initiation of the process of illness causation. Obviously, however, causes also have causes (#1b), a concept that has recently received attention from the social determinants of health perspective (Braveman and Gottlieb 2014). Also, many kinds of illness have multiple kinds of causes (#1c). One simple example includes genetic disorders that have multiple different gene aberrations as a possible "root cause," such as autism spectrum disorders (Gaugler et al. 2014).

Philosophers have contrasted what they call *causal productivity* or *production* with *causal propagation*, the influence of events at one place and time on events at another place and time (Salmon 1993), or *relevance/difference-making*, the idea that a cause can make a difference to an effect without producing it (Glennan 2011). Since the etiological process is a *biological* process, the inducer has to have the capacity to start the biological chain of events.[8] In the biosciences, this capacity is conceived of as the logical and biological capability of a signal to be propagated in a biological process.[9]

Consider, for example, one review article in the *Journal of Experimental & Clinical Cancer Research* is entitled, "Dual effect of oxidative stress on leukemia cancer induction and treatment" (Udensi and Tchounwou 2014). The paper describes the double-edged-sword-like effects of oxidative stress (OS), mainly in the form of an overabundance of reactive oxygen species (ROS) in tissues, on body cells in both pro- and anticancer biological processes. The authors use the term *induction* in a causal way, as illustrated by the following examples:

- "Many chemotherapeutic drugs have been shown to exert their biologic activity through *induction* of OS in affected cells."
- "Endogenous DNA damage demonstrates the genotoxic, carcinogenic, and mutations *induction* properties of ROS."
- "A traditional Chinese medicine, Mylabris, exerts its anticancer effects through *induction* of oxidative stress."

In all these examples, induction is a form of causation that is defined as the initiation of a mechanism, the starting of a process, and the generation of a biological phenomenon, mainly *inside the body*. In epidemiology, the induction kind of causation is conceptualized as the beginning of the disease process by induction of the bodily disease causation process from *outside the body*. Examples are exposure to radiation or tobacco smoke, which induces changes in skin and lung cells, respectively, which demarcates the beginning of the skin/lung cancer pathogenesis process. In philosophy, this kind of causation has been called "primary cause" (Bunge 1979:49), "efficient cause [,] or stimulus condition" (Mumford and Anjum 2011a:33).

The idea that mechanisms play a prominent role in etiological processes offers room for the view that different parts of such mechanisms have different functions in that they contribute to the etiological process in different ways. The suggestion to move from concepts of illness causation to the concept of contribution to illness goes back to Severinsen's discussion of disease mechanism as a basis for disease classification systems, in which he states that

> if asked to give an objective answer to what the mechanism or the causal structure behind a disease is, one could argue that there are many "causal factors" in a complex structure of causes, and that, in most cases, those factors are neither sufficient nor necessary, but only contributory. (Severinsen 2001:322)

7.3.3 Modification

John Stuart Mill (1806–1873) coined the phrase "composition of causes" for cases "in which the joint effect of several causes is identical with the sum of their separate effects" (Mill 1856:Chapter v, §1). In cases, however, where

> a concurrence of causes takes place which calls into action new laws, bearing no analogy to any that we can trace in the separate operation of the causes, the new laws may supersede one portion of the previous laws but coexist with another portion, and may even compound the effect of those previous laws with their own. (Mill 1856:Chapter v, §2)

This comes close to what statisticians call *interaction*, what epidemiologists think of as *effect modification*, and what psychologists mean when they use the term *moderation* (Figure 7.3, in particular 2b–d). In epidemiology, the concept of effect modification, a.k.a., *effect measure modification* (Rothman, Greenland, and Lash 2008b), is rather important.

Consider the following situation. In a large randomized trial including almost 40,000 healthy women, 45 years or older, designed to test the hypothesis that low-dose aspirin prevents cardiovascular disease in women, a prominent statistically significant protective effect of aspirin on major cardiovascular events (risk reduction by 26%) was identified in women 65 years or older, while no effect was observed among women 64 years or younger (Ridker et al. 2005). This is an example of effect modification by age: an effect is observed in one age group but not in another. Obviously, such results have direct implications for interventionalists. While it may seem best to prescribe aspirin to women 65 or older, but not to younger women, potential risks must be weighed against the benefits. In this case, in the age group 65 years or older, 44 fewer myocardial infarctions or deaths were seen, but aspirin use came with 16 more cases of gastrointestinal hemorrhage.

One particularly interesting kind of modification is *inhibition* (Figure 7.3, #2a):

- "[Substance X] has been reported to exert its therapeutic action against APL cancer through *induction* of cell differentiation via mechanisms that include degradation of PML-RARA gene and *inhibition* of arachidonic acid metabolic pathway in other cancer cells." (Udensi and Tchounwou 2014:8)
- "Application of antioxidant principles may illicit same effect [*sic*], for example *inhibition* of intracellular antioxidants such as GSH and heme oxygenase-1 (HO-1)." (p. 10)

Inhibitors of causal processes can remove the cause entirely or partially block its immediate effects to various degrees. They can also interrupt the pathomechanism or slow it down. Thus, inhibitors can result in the prevention of illness or in other, more gradual changes in illness occurrence, for example, by slowing down the etiological process. One objection to this proposal would be that process inhibition cannot count as a *causal* contributor because it does not contribute to the *occurrence* of a health phenomenon, other than potentially *decreasing* the risk of the outcome to occur. This is what protective risk factors do; they are associated with a reduced risk of the outcome under investigation. Inhibition does not contribute to the merely qualitative aspect of illness *occurrence*, at least not in the sense of contributing to its occurrence among individuals who do not have it. However, their potential to reduce illness severity or even prevent illness occurrence renders inhibitors *very* important contributors to illness etiology that we should be interested in at least as much as we are interested in root causes.

Another objection would be that inhibition is by definition not a contribution to the process that it interferes with, because it represents a separate process, that is, that of process inhibition. It would be taking the easy way out to say that inhibitory factors are part of the etiological story of a certain illness, because finding such a factor is mouthwatering for epidemiologists and biomedical scientists because they now have a new target for intervention. Hold on to the notion that inhibition is a kind of explanatory part of the etiological process, not so much because it helps explain *why* the health outcome occurs, but because interference helps explain why the outcome occurs in the form and magnitude it does, but not in a different one.

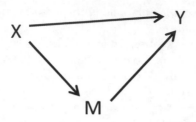

Figure 7.4 Partial mediation of X's effect on Z.

7.3.4 Mediation

It is arguably self-evident that mediation is contribution. Mediators (Figure 7.3, #3a,b) are intermediate factors in the form $X > M > Y$. In this scenario, X causes Y, but only indirectly so, that is, by causing M, which in turn causes Y. Thus, we say the effect of X on Y is wholly mediated by M when X cannot lead to Y except through mediation. Mediation can also be *partial*, when X causes Y directly as well as via mediation by M (Figure 7.4).[10]

Woodward distinguishes between two notions of cause. The first is the notion of a *total cause,* which is a cause if and only if an intervention on it and on no other variables results in a nonzero total effect on the outcome (Woodward 2003:50). In contrast, a *contributing cause* is a *direct or indirect* cause that has a nonzero effect on the outcome by influencing a *direct* cause of the outcome while all variables that are not on the causal pathway are kept constant.[11] Per Woodward, direct causes are always contributors, while some contributors may also be indirect. In our current context, all mediators are contributors, because they are all considered direct causes.[12]

Taken together, I think that induction, modification, and mediation qualify as modes of contribution to stories of illness occurrence in ways that render them helpful in understanding the etiology of illness. If nothing else, this makes them valuable items in comprehensive etiological explanations.

Given the heterogeneity of contributors displayed in Figure 7.2, I feel the need to reiterate that contributors *include* causes and all other kinds of factors that somehow contribute to illness occurrence. In this sense, a contributor is anything that transmits a mark. Of course, we need some kind of justification to include or exclude contributors in etiological explanations. This is the topic for the next and last chapter, where my thinking about *explanatory coherence* as a way to create such comprehensive etiological explanations is outlined.

8 ETIOLOGICAL COHERENCE

8.1 INTRODUCTION

In Chapter 3, etiological explanations were introduced, and it was argued that they fall under a pluralist concept (in Chapter 4). Introduced was the kind of explanation envisaged by the central argument of the Russo–Williamson thesis (RWT), who talk about evidence of difference-making (association) and evidence of mechanism in support of causal claims in the health sciences (Chapter 5). My take on this is that, instead of RWT kind of evidence, we need evidence that supports etiological explanations. In Chapter 6, it was proposed that etiological explanations are explanations of a biological trajectory from causes via pathomechanisms to disease and that, therefore, etiological explanations explain a process. In comparison to explanations of mechanisms, where the focus is on components of mechanisms and their relationships, process explanations focus on the sequence of events in the etiological story. In Chapter 7, it was argued that including background conditions and other contributors such as mediators and modifiers can render etiological explanations of illness occurrence more comprehensive, which is considered an explanatory virtue.

In this chapter, first, some brief, overarching thoughts about *explanatory coherentism* are offered. This philosophical framework might be a good fit for the design of comprehensive etiological explanations (Section 8.1). Section 8.2 is based on a paper previously published in the *American Journal of Epidemiology* (Dammann 2018). It is an attempt to connect Hill's viewpoints (introduced in Section 2.5.2 and expanded upon later) with concepts from Ted Poston's book, *Reason and Explanation: A Defense of Explanatory Coherentism* (Poston 2014). Poston's theory of explanatory coherentism is well suited as a tool for etiological explanation in the health sciences, particularly in epidemiology. As a caveat, Poston's theory is not one of *explanation* but of *explanatory justification*. It explicates why explanatory coherentism can deliver justification to believe certain claims.

Coherence has not only played a role in epidemiology as one of Hill's viewpoints, it can also provide background theory for the development of explanatory systems by integrating epidemiological evidence with a diversity of other error-independent scientific data. Computational formalization of Hill's viewpoints in an explanatory coherentist framework would provide an excellent starting point for a formal epistemological (knowledge-theoretical) project designed to improve causal explanation in the health sciences. As an example, Paul Thagard's ECHO System is introduced and my responses to possible objections to my proposal are offered.

In Section 8.3. we dig a little deeper into what Hill's intentions might have been and flesh out my proposal that his heuristics make for an interesting explanatory coherentist framework for etiological explanations. In what follows, the foundations for that proposal are set out.

8.2 HILL'S HEURISTICS AND EXPLANATORY COHERENTISM IN EPIDEMIOLOGY

8.2.1 Introduction

This section is a response to two invitations. The first comes from philosopher Alex Broadbent, who asks epidemiologists to take an explanatory stance in the causal interpretation of measures of association (Broadbent 2013). The second is from epidemiologist Alfredo Morabia, who suggests that Hill's viewpoints (Hill 1965) cannot be traced back to the work of classic philosophers of causality, Hume and Mill, but constitute a *sui generis* approach to causal discovery, "which still awaits its philosophers" (Morabia 2013).

Ted Poston's version of explanatory coherentism (Poston 2014) is introduced. Next, Hill's concept of coherence is revisited. Then, the idea that the two could be brought together in a formalized analysis software, such as Thagard's ECHO system, is considered. Finally, the position against three main objections from the foundationalist perspective, from the perspective of the potential outcomes approach (POA) (Glass et al. 2013), and from the "computational skeptic" angle is defended.

8.2.2 Explanatory coherentism

Philosopher Ted Poston probably did not have epidemiologists in mind as a target audience for his book *Reason and Explanation: A Defense of Explanatory Coherentism* (Poston 2014). Still, his theory appears to be relevant to epidemiology as a potential way to semiformalize the kind of approach to causal explanation represented by Hill's viewpoints. Ken Rothman and coauthors suggest that for Hill, "causal inference is a subjective matter of degree of personal belief, certainty, or conviction" and that "this view is precisely that of subjective Bayesian statistics" (Rothman et al. 2008a, 2008b, 2008c). Epidemiologists should be interested in theories such as Poston's because explanatory coherentism is the justification of a statement by showing that it is part of an explanatory system, which is internally coherent and externally better than alternative systems. It deserves mention that the idea, to require not just a good causal explanation, but one that is better than others, is not Poston's, but is based on a concept in philosophy of science called "inference to the best explanation" (Harman 1965; Lipton 2004), which is essentially a method of eliminating alternative explanations until one, purportedly the best, remains unchallenged. A more detailed discussion of this idea goes far beyond the scope of this chapter.

Poston's theory holds that the normative position of a person's reasoning is defined by how that person *explains* what is going on in herself and the world around her, and that she justifies her beliefs by fitting them into a "virtuous explanatory system" (as defined later) that is better than relevant alternative systems. She gathers data about facts, puts them in context, compares her explanatory system to others, and considers her beliefs justified if her belief system turns out to beat all competitors.

Naturally, not all agree that such a view can replace one that favors the truth over coherence. In philosophy, this camp is called the "foundationalists," whose claim is that coherentism and other nonfoundationalist theories fail because the world cannot rest on the back of a turtle that rests on the back of a turtle that rests on the back of a turtle …, and it is turtles all the way down.[1] Foundationalists hold that there is one last turtle all the way down, and it stands on a foundation that is *not* based on any inference.

Poston offers a theory of justification that incorporates the notions of explanation, coherence, and contrast. He states that one "has justification for believing p if and only if p is a member of a sufficiently virtuous explanatory system, E, and E is more virtuous than any competing system E'" (Poston 2014:87). At this point, let's define two crucial elements of Poston's earlier statement.

First, being a member of an explanatory system means being an item that explains (*explanans*) or that is to be explained (*explanandum*). Second, for this explanatory system to be "sufficiently virtuous" means, in Poston's framework, to be "sufficiently conservative, simple, or great in power." An explanation is conservative if we always have a situation in which we have *some* background knowledge that helps defending our belief in the truth of a statement even without additional evidence. An explanation is simple if it involves fewer components than competitor explanatory systems. Finally, an explanation is powerful if it explains a diversity of phenomena.

Second, all of these involve contrastive evaluation of explanatory systems, and evaluation in comparison to alternatives. This notion is derived from inference to the best explanation, the idea that explaining why risk factor A but not risk factor B causes outcome O is better than just explaining why A causes O. Of course, inference to the best explanation also has noncontrastive characteristics, which are of lesser importance in our present context than contrastivity.

In the final chapter of his book, Poston shows that explanationism and Bayesianism are compatible – a connection that is in keeping with Rothman et al.'s link between causal inference and subjective Bayesianism, as well as Lipton's defense of the compatibility of inference to the best explanation and Bayesian inference (Lipton 2004). Explanation and its virtues represent the scientific tradition of using the notions of law, causation, and explanation to argue for the superiority of some hypothesis over others. Bayesianism is a purely formal model that does not incorporate these notions. Poston shows how the two views of inductive inference fit together and in fact supplement each other – an observation that is welcome to those who advocate for the integration of Bayesian thinking in meta-analysis (Sutton and Abrams 2001), genetic (Wilson et al. 2010), spatial (Lawson 2012), and clinical epidemiology (Luthra 2015), as well as in causal inference (Williamson 2005) and causal theory building (Sloman and Lagnado 2015).

Poston's theory is well suited for causal explanation in epidemiology for two closely related reasons. First, coherence is one of the classical Hill viewpoints (Hill 1965).

Second, Poston's work can provide background theory for the development of explanatory systems. Within epidemiology, it can serve as one way to decide among competing explanatory systems. In a transdisciplinary context, it can help integrate epidemiological evidence with evidence from independent sources, such as basic laboratory science, interventional trials, and postmarketing data.

8.2.3 Explanation *in silico*

A particularly intriguing way to use Hill's heuristics as explanatory virtues would be to integrate it with a computational coherence assessment system. For example, Paul Thagard has developed computational models of coherence and integrated them with aspects of scientific communication into a consensus model of scientific discourse (Thagard 2000). Thagard and colleagues have formalized his theory of explanatory coherence (Thagard 2000, 2004, 2006, 2007) in the computational model ECHO. The algorithm accommodates seven principles[2]:

E1. *Symmetry*: Explanatory coherence is a symmetrical relation. That is, two propositions P and Q cohere with each other equally.

E2. *Explanation*: (a) A hypothesis coheres with what it explains, which can either be evidence or another hypothesis; (b) hypotheses that together explain some other proposition cohere with each other; and (c) the more hypotheses it takes to explain something, the lower the degree of coherence.

E3. *Analogy*: Similar hypotheses that explain similar pieces of evidence cohere with each other.

E4. *Data priority*: Propositions that describe the results of observations have a degree of acceptability on their own.

E5. *Contradiction*: Contradictory propositions are incoherent with each other.

E6. *Competition*: If P and Q both explain a proposition, and if P and Q are not explanatorily connected, then P and Q are incoherent with each other. (P and Q are explanatorily connected if one explains the other or if together they explain something.)

E7. *Acceptance*: The acceptability of a proposition in a system of propositions depends on its coherence with them. (Thagard 2006)

As an example, Thagard modeled the coherence of the decision-making process in the courtroom (Thagard 2004). He fed ECHO information available to jurors in the notorious case of Martha von Bülow, who was found unconscious in 1980 and remained in a coma until her death in 2008. Her husband Claus was found guilty of assault with intent to murder in 1982. He appealed and was acquitted in a second trial. Thagard successfully demonstrates that ECHO arrives at the same results: "For the first trial, ECHO ends up accepting the hypothesis that Claus injected [his wife] with insulin, but for the second trial ECHO ends up rejecting it" (Thagard 2004).

It is possible to design a software similar to ECHO in which Hill's viewpoints are incorporated as explanatory virtues. Each one of ECHO's requirements listed earlier can be viewed as a decision point; Hill's viewpoints are nothing else. Once fed with pertinent epidemiological and other bioscientific data, such a program could function as a decision-tree-like algorithm, which is a computational method that has regained importance in the context of machine learning (Kelleher, Mac Namee, and D'Arcy 2015). It would be possible to validate such semiformal software in comparison to informal current analyses of causal explanation, for example, of the causal association between Zika virus and birth defects (Frank, Faber, and Stark 2016; Rasmussen et al. 2016). Due to space limitations, the semantics of such software cannot be fully developed, but here are a few desiderata: the input of evidence data should include text-mining strategies moderated by human expertise; a modifiable weighing of Hill's heuristics should be included; and the software designers would need to be creative in translating Hill's open-ended questions into the rigid syntax of a programming language in order to retain the overarching explanatory intention of Hill's viewpoints.

In this section, it was proposed that a computational explanatory coherentist tool for decision-making might be helpful in the overall project of bringing causal explanation together with complex systems thinking in epidemiology (Galea, Riddle, and Kaplan 2010; Marshall and Galea 2015; Pearce and Merletti 2006). Discussed in the next section is how this proposal is aligned with Hill's viewpoints.

8.2.4 Hill's coherence

Since their initial publication, Hill's viewpoints have been extensively discussed in the epidemiological and philosophical literature (Höfler 2005, 2006; Ioannidis 2015; Morabia 1991, 2013; Phillips and Goodman 2004, 2006; Rothman 1988; Rothman and Greenland 2005; Thygesen, Andersen, and Andersen 2005; Ward 2009a, 2009b; Worrall 2011). The overall agreement appears to be that although they cannot prove causation, they can still be useful. Phillips and Goodman put it in a nutshell: "Hill's famous considerations are thus both over-interpreted by those who would use them as criteria and under-appreciated as lessons in basic scientific thinking" (Phillips and Goodman 2006).

It is not my intention to discuss all nine viewpoints in detail in this chapter. Instead, the focus is on Hill's view of coherence and how it can support causal claims in epidemiology and beyond.

An explanatory coherentist reconstruction of Hill's viewpoints is in keeping with his intention to offer a tool for decision-making. Interpreting Hill's approach as motivated by a contrastive explanatory stance is aligned with reflection on cases from the literature where his heuristics are used as explanatory virtues in causal explanations.

First, Hill's heuristics can be viewed as "explanatory virtues" that are used to assess the relative worth of competing causal explanations; the greater their contrastive explanatory virtue, the more we are justified to assume causation. Hill was convinced that his viewpoints can be useful by means of finding alternative explanations that are better than causation (Hill 1965:298).

Hill suggests that causal claims can be strengthened by coherent evidence from multiple observations and gives as an example the coherence of the claim that causally relates smoking and lung cancer with observations such as concomitant increase of both exposure and outcome over time, as well as sex differences in both smoking behavior and mortality (p. 298).

In this part of his explication of "coherence," Hill refers to evidence from *within* epidemiological research. He argues that an association between smoking and lung disease that can be detected by conducting a cohort study should not be easily contradicted by results obtained in, for example, an ecological study, which (as in his earlier example) would yield population-level data for both smoking and lung disease over time without reference to person-level data.

Second, interpreting Hill's heuristics as explanatory virtues appreciates their value as "countervailing evidence limiters." Looking at possible competitor explanations in light of Hill's heuristics increases the likelihood that the index causal claim remains at the top of the list of explanations, at least until one such competitor explanation turns out to be more coherent.

Third, epidemiological evidence in support of causal claims may be strong if supported by multiple observations, but it is even stronger if supported by multiple *different kinds* of observation. Hill's viewpoints ask for error-independent evidence (Claveau 2012), the explanatory benefit carried by multiple sources of evidence that cannot be invalidated for the same reason. In brief, two or more pieces of evidence are error-independent if the failure of one does not affect the stability of the other. In our context, if epidemiological evidence turns out to be false, it would not render otherwise coherent biological evidence incorrect, and vice versa. Thus, evidence becomes stronger "if multiple, (more or less) error-independent, evidential elements support the same claim" (Claveau 2012:812).

Hill suggests further that epidemiological evidence should not be in conflict with background information about the *biological mechanism* of the disease. As an example, he refers to histological abnormalities in the lung and the isolation of carcinogenic substances from cigarette smoke (Hill 1965:298).

While some philosophers of science think that in order to make causal claims in the health sciences, one needs evidence of both difference-making (statistical associations) and evidence of mechanism (Russo and Williamson 2007b), some of us hold that having both kinds of evidence may be sufficient but certainly not necessary for successful causal claims (Broadbent 2011; Fiorentino and Dammann 2015). In this regard, Hill remains completely neutral by explicitly denying that finding evidence in support of his viewpoints should be considered necessary to establish causal claims.

8.2.5 Objections and rebuttal

Among the possible objections to this proposal are objections against coherentism in general, against Hill's viewpoints as a method for causal explanation, and against the idea to formalize Hill's heuristics.

Objections against coherentism come, for example, from anticoherentist Erik Olsson, who writes (with direct reference to Thagard's version of coherentism) that "there is no way to define a useful informative concept of degree of coherence such that more coherence implies a higher likelihood of truth *ceteris paribus*" (Olsson 2005). This argument, although probably considered a strong one by foundationalists, is beside the point in our current scenario, simply because we are not searching for truth *ceteris paribus*, but for an explanation that leads to more fruitful action than competitors. Moreover, foundationalism has yet to deliver a method to infer truth from observed data. Note that switching to the fruitful action criterion does not invalidate Olsson's objection; it merely moves the goalposts into a pragmatist direction. It remains to be shown whether and how it is possible to establish degrees of coherence. Perhaps by allocating relative weights to Hill's viewpoints – while one (temporality) is being considered a *sine qua non* (Rothman et al. 2008a, 2008b, 2008c), another (analogy) we can live without, although its presence in the body of evidence would certainly add to the overall coherence of the system to be explained.

Perhaps the strongest opposition might come from advocates of the POA, who consider their approach worthy of the appellation "modern approach," while Hill's viewpoints are implicitly demoted to the status of "classic framework" (Glass et al. 2013). Glass and colleagues note that

> (Hill's) classic framework was developed to identify the causes of diseases and […] has proven useful […], but does not reflect the current, more clearly articulated view of causal processes. Additionally, the guidelines used to evaluate evidence have not changed for decades. (Glass et al. 2013)

There are no less than four points to be argued with this statement.

First, it is incorrect that Hill's goal was to "identify causes." Instead, he wanted to offer help with contrastive explanation ("is there any other way of explaining the set of facts before us" [Hill 1953]). Yes, contrastive explanation can help identify causes via inference to the best explanation (Lipton 2004). However, Hill's heuristics help by providing evidence in support of the inference part, not by criteria for what the best explanation should entail. Glass and colleagues write that the fundamental problem with causal inference from observational data is confounding and that one needs to bend over backward to adjust for all possible measured confounders by using appropriate methods like matching, stratification, propensity scores, g-estimation, and so forth. Those who deal with confounders for a living will ask what has become of residual confounding. The term is conspicuously absent from Glass et al.'s paper. Either the authors forgot to discuss it (unlikely), or they do not consider residual confounding an important issue (even more unlikely). Douglas Weed wrote some time ago that "causation cannot be seen. Causation cannot be proven. […] Nor can causation be made certain. It is, at best, an expert's judgment, at worst, an expert's guess" (Weed 2008). That is, I think, what Hill had in mind: to support experts' admittedly fallible judgements by offering a set of questions they can ask themselves to ponder before we "pass from this observed *association* to a verdict of *causation*" (Hill 1965). That future semiformal ECHO-like algorithms might contribute to the generation of fair verdicts and judgements that are better than those arrived at via free-floating nonformal assessment.

Second, Hill's viewpoints are useful despite their fallibility. More than half a century after their publication, they are still given room in epidemiology textbooks, for a reason: They help epidemiologists to evaluate and weigh the available evidence for and against causal hypotheses, as in recent publications on Zika virus infection and birth defects (Lipton 2004).

Third, Hill's viewpoints should be able to take care of causal *processes*. I am also not sure in what way our view of causal processes is more clearly articulated now than in 1965. Concepts of illness causation have included the notion of a biological process in the 1960s as much as they do now, and the idea of an etiological process was well established in 1949, as evidenced in a case report on methemoglobinemia and Minnesota well water, in reference to the kinds of etiological processes that epidemiologists try to disentangle:

> The father of the first infant [suggested a] reaction between the well water and the soy bean preparation used in the baby's formula [...] analysis of the well water showed a high nitrate content. Thus the etiologic process was discovered. (Bosch et al. 1950)

Fourth, it is true that the guidelines have not changed since their initial publication in 1965. There is no reason to assume that they should be changed just because they were published half a century ago. They have stood the test of time for a reason: they are useful. Moreover, the nature of illness causation has not changed much over the past 50 years. What has changed are our concepts of causal inference and explanation, but adapting our interpretation of Hill's heuristics accordingly may be insufficient to maintain their value for epidemiological reasoning.

Why should the POA be any better than "modern" reconstructions of Hill's apparently rather successful viewpoints? Observational data, even if stratified and analyzed according to the presence or absence of hypothetical interventions, are still observational. Why should data from hypothetical interventions be better than observational data if even data from *real* interventions, such as randomized trials, might not necessarily be epistemologically superior (Cartwright 2010; Worrall 2007)? The POA and Hill's approach are *different*, in that the POA is a *quantitative* method to extract causal information from observed data, primarily from one particular dataset to which the approach is applied. In contrast, Hill's framework is a *qualitative* approach, integrating information from multiple sources, not just one study. Thus, the two approaches are not mutually exclusive; to the contrary, they are supplementing each other.

There are doubts that the POA should be considered superior and become the sole standard approach to causal explanation in epidemiology. Vandenbroucke, Broadbent, and Pearce wrote that they "feel (the POA) would damage the discipline if it became the dominant paradigm" (Vandenbroucke, Broadbent, and Pearce 2016). Their critique is addressed to a particular version of the POA that they call the restricted POA, that is, a POA restricted by the rejection of (1) manipulations that are not humanly feasible and thus not interesting to epidemiologists, and (2) causal claims that do not allow for predictions under hypothetical scenarios. A full discussion of their comprehensive discussion is far beyond the scope of this chapter; suffice it to say that Vandenbroucke et al. cogently argue against the notion that the tools of the restricted POA "are the only or even the best tools for assessing causality" and are in favor of "a pragmatic pluralism about concepts of causality" (ibid.) Indeed, the integration of multiple kinds of evidence in the search for actionable causes of illness is a central characteristic of our current epidemiological thinking, albeit still without a formal theoretical framework for knowledge integration.

Another objection would be to say that a computational approach to a coherentist version of Hill's framework as explanatory virtues is unlikely to be better than Hill's framework as is. My response to this is: we do not know this until we have tried. Thus, my proposal to explore the value of computational coherentist tools for causal thinking in epidemiology and biomedicine is justified. I also suggest that theories such as Poston's and Thagard's would provide an excellent starting point for such a project.

8.3 POSTSCRIPT – HILL'S ETIOLOGICAL COHERENTISM[3]

8.3.1 Introduction

The seminal paper by Sir Austin Bradford Hill (1965) on causal inference in previous chapters.[4] In the previous section, development has begun on a framework that conceives of Hill's viewpoints as an explanatory coherentist system. This proposal goes beyond coherence as one of Hill's nine viewpoints.[5] Instead, explanatory coherence can be seen as the theory behind Hill's viewpoints, or what others have called "aspects" (Ward 2009b), "values" (Poole 2001), or "considerations" (Höfler 2006).

In this section, response is given to Broadbent's invitation to "advance beyond Hill's viewpoints [by asking] how good evidence needs to be before it warrants a causal inference" (Broadbent 2013:69). But before going there, in Section 8.3.2 we ask what Hill's conception of illness causation may have been in the first place and what he may have wanted to present, if not criteria for causation. He was clearly interested in developing a heuristic for the *justification of decisions to act*. It seems to be explicit in his paper that Hill suggested his viewpoints with *action* in mind. However, Hill knew that he would have to pay a price for getting to a justification of action: he would have to replace the idea of causal inference based on solid criteria with the idea of inference based on heuristics (viewpoints, aspects, etc.), thereby embracing the epistemological intricacies of inductive fallibility.

We also provide an answer to the question of what Hill's criteria have to offer if they are neither a checklist of characteristics for those who seek a "yes" or "no" answer to the causal question, nor a continuous measure of how strong the evidence is in support of such a "yes" or "no" answer. In Section 8.3.3, it is proposed that Hill's viewpoints are explanatory virtues in an explanatory coherentist system (Poston 2014) of statements that can be compared to alternative systems. In recognition of my space constraints in this chapter, three topics are only briefly addressed that will remain to be explored in depth at a later time (Section 8.3.4). First, future work needs to outline in what ways and why there is disagreement with Poston's notion of explanatory primitiveness; second, it remains to be shown whether and how my Hill-Poston-inspired view of etiological explanations resonates with unificationist models of explanation (Friedman 1974; Kitcher 1989); and third, my observation that Hill's viewpoints are metaphysically heterogeneous needs to be outlined in more detail (Russo and Williamson 2007b; Thygesen, Andersen, and Andersen 2005), which further improves their explanatory virtue by providing what Claveau has called *error-independent evidence* (Claveau 2012).

8.3.2 Hill's heuristics as justification for action

It is interesting that nowhere in his paper does Hill write anything about his perception of what illness causation is – he does not offer a definition. He writes that he does not have the "wish, nor the skill, to embark upon a philosophical discussion of the meaning of 'causation'" (Hill 1965:295). By saying this, Hill makes it clear that his approach is not guided by *metaphysical* considerations. Instead, he states his *epistemological* problem a few lines below: "The decisive question is whether the frequency of the undesirable event B will be influenced by the environmental feature A" (ibid.). Thus, Hill's question is about *causation as influence*. As such, it is a question about the relationship between the two sets of characteristics, one being a constellation of risk factors that, taken together, appear to be responsible for illness occurrence by exerting an influence, and the other being the set of characteristics that defines the illness under consideration. In this context, it seems that causal inference is about what we think we should think about relationships between characteristics of etiological systems we have before us. It is about what beliefs we think we are justified to hold about the relationship between risk factors and illness occurrence. To make that decision (whether we think we are justified or not), we need explanations, based on observed data and their coherence among each other and with prior knowledge.

There is no intent to add much to the discussion of whether or not the Hill "criteria" are, in fact, criteria in the sense of necessary and sufficient conditions. Many years of debate about this in the epidemiological literature suggests that there is no such thing as hard criteria for illness causation. But what are Hill's "criteria," if not criteria?

Hill stated in no uncertain terms that the causal knowledge we are to gain from his viewpoints is needed to guide our *actions*. He writes that

> before deducing "causation" and taking action, we shall not invariably have to sit around awaiting the results of that research. (Hill 1965:295)

This brief quote from Hill's paper's first page anticipates what he devotes a whole section to on its last, entitled "The case for action." In that section, Hill makes some important statements worthy of mention. He writes that

> the evidence is there to be judged on its merits and the judgment (in that sense) should be utterly independent of what hangs upon it – or who hangs because of it. (Hill 1965:300)

Still, he asserts that in occupational medicine (his own field of research), action is often the objective. He thinks that once the

> operative cause and [...] deleterious effect [have been identified] we shall wish to intervene to abolish or reduce death or disease. (ibid.)

Hill also had *good results* in mind. He was goal oriented, and his goal was to inform decisions about actions by means of the best possible causal inference, defined by yielding the best possible results. In pragmatist terms, we may call a result good if it helps improve the human condition. In the health sciences, success of good inferential thinking is measured in terms of successful public health interventions that prevent illness, medical interventions that make patients better, and surgical interventions that increase and improve survival. But how good must evidence be before it warrants causal inference (Broadbent 2013:69)? We come back to this question later.

Despite his enthusiasm for causal inference in the service of action, Hill knows that

> All scientific work is incomplete – whether it be observational or experimental. All scientific work is liable to be upset or modified by advancing knowledge. That does not confer upon us a freedom to ignore the knowledge we already have, or to postpone the action that it appears to demand at a given time. (Hill 1965:300)

Hill's quest is an epistemological one, a search for a (more or less) formal framework for inquiry that helps generate knowledge, a set of rules to distinguish between association and causation. If viewed from his action-oriented perspective, one could think of his suggestions as being motivated by the search for a set of reasons that would persuade others to take action.[6] His viewpoints can be seen as points of guidance toward evidence that justifies action.

However, Hill knows that the kind of knowledge generation he is after is not rule based. Therefore, he makes sure his readers understand the limitations of his "aspects" and writes that

> in asking for very strong evidence I would, however, repeat emphatically that this does not imply crossing every "t," and swords with every critic, before we act. All scientific work is incomplete – whether it be observational or experimental. All scientific work is liable to be upset or modified by advancing knowledge. (ibid.)

Hill's argument resonates well with the commonplace notion that there is no such thing as complete and persistent certainty, in science or, arguably, anywhere else.

This perspective gives rise to an interesting thought. While Hill shies away from the concept of criteria and moves toward the less stringent heuristic of viewpoints instead, he does not leave us with the impression that he considers this a weakness of his proposal. To the contrary: In the last paragraph of his paper, Hill writes hopefully and in a rather upbeat fashion:

> Who knows, asked Robert Browning, but the world may end tonight? True, but on available evidence most of us make ready to commute on the 8.30 next day. (ibid.)

It seems as if Hill was confident that his viewpoints would do a reasonable job *even without being criteria*. This suggests that *we can live with uncertainty* in the health sciences and still do a good job. Just like every one of us makes sense of our everyday lives in rather inexact ways,[7] it seems likely, based on the successes of medicine and public health over the past century, that *we do not need criteria* and that Hill's viewpoints have done a pretty good job as helpers toward better, albeit imperfect, causal inference and explanation, justified actions, and improved health.

Based on these considerations, for Hill, the meaning of his viewpoints was, more or less, their function as pointers toward aspects of an observed association that would make it *potentially useful* as a target for intervention. In other words, Hill's viewpoints are characteristics of an association that, if being acted upon, is likely to yield useful *results*.[8] At least partially, it is also a goal-oriented, "functional approach to causation, (…) that takes as its point of departure the idea that causal information and reasoning are sometimes useful or functional in the sense of serving various goals and purposes that we have" (Woodward 2014).

In summary, Hill's heuristics are not criteria, and the decision that an observed association between risk factor and illness is causal has no foundation in some sort of criteria. What Hill's viewpoints offer, however, is help in explaining illness occurrence – as argued next.

8.3.3 Hill's viewpoints as backbone of coherent etiological explanations

Beyond providing justification for action, Hill was also interested in *explaining* disease occurrence, in providing etiological explanations.[9] Etiological explanations are scientific explanations. Scientific explanations provide pieces of information (explanantia) about phenomena (explananda) that increase our knowledge about why and how the explananda come about (Woodward 2017). Coherentism comes in three forms, each one with different goals. The coherence theory *of truth* "states that the truth of any (true) proposition consists in its coherence with some specified set of propositions" (Young 2018). The coherence theory *of justification* holds that "a belief or set of beliefs is justified, or justifiably held, just in case the belief coheres with a set of beliefs, the set forms a coherent system or some variation on these themes."

The third kind of coherence theory, *explanatory coherence,* holds that evidential coherence adds explanatory force to an explanation; "it is what makes it an explanation, not just another fact."[10] In this view, having credible support by multiple pieces of evidence from multiple sources for an explanation would make that explanation better than another one that is supported by only one or two pieces of evidence from only one or two sources. This kind of coherence does not support truth statements, and it does not bear on someone's justification to believe or act in such and such a way, but it does help distinguish between, for example, good explanations and *better* explanations. An explanation is good if it offers a credible set of pieces of evidence that support it; an explanation is better if it offers a credible *and coherent* set of pieces of evidence that support it. Note that it is not the amount of evidence but the coherence among pieces of evidence that makes it better than incoherent ones. However, coherent explanations can be improved by providing *more* data that are coherent with previously available coherent data. Taken together, we can show how Hill's heuristics and Poston's explanatory coherentism can reach across the aisle between coherence theories of explanation on the one hand and coherence theories of justification on the other hand.

Poston suggests that "a subject's propositional justification for any claim is a matter of how that claim fits into a virtuous explanatory system that beats relevant competitors" (Poston 2014:2).

In other words, Poston offers an *explanationist theory of justification* (Ex-J):

S has justification for believing p if and only if p is a member of a sufficiently virtuous explanatory system, *E*, and *E* is more virtuous than any competing system *E'*. (Poston 2014:87)

This is a coherentist approach to justification that is based on explanatory systems. It tells us that someone is justified to believe a claim or hypothesis, namely, if it is part of a coherent explanatory system that is more virtuous than its competitors are. Thus, Ex-J has two conditions for justification, *proper membership* in a sufficiently virtuous coherent explanatory system and *superior virtuosity* of that explanatory system over competitors. Obviously, both conditions require further clarification in order to make the relevant decisions when a new p_i becomes available. For the first, we need to specify what qualifies as good evidence and what qualifies as sufficient virtuosity. For the second one, we need to decide what qualifies as greater virtuosity. For example, does the virtuosity of *E* increase with an increasing number of its members $p_1 \dots p_n$ that qualify as being justified to be believed in? In that case, having evidence for the *E* makes it a stronger competitor against any weaker explanatory system *E'*. Only if *E* wins over *E'* is the view justified that the etiological explanation captured by *E* is better than another etiological explanation *E'*. Still, Ex-J does not tell us anything about what exactly an explanatory system is, how we come to know that it is sufficiently virtuous, and how we find out whether it is more virtuous than other systems, let alone *any* other system. However, Hill's heuristics can be used to make the decision whether any new data fulfill both the *proper membership* and *superior virtuosity* requirements.[11]

To do this, we need to proceed as in the following example. First, we need to apply the first condition of Ex-J, *proper membership*, to an etiological explanation à la Bradford Hill. Let p_i be any one of Hill's viewpoints $p_1 \dots p_9$ and etiological explanation *E* be the union of all viewpoints $[p_1 \dots p_i]$ for which we have good evidence that we consider sufficiently virtuous. According to Ex-J's first requirement, subject S is justified to believe that p_i if and only if it is a member of *E*. Consider a situation in which we are interested in the etiology of skin cancer and we already have evidence that strongly supports Hill's viewpoint #1, *strength* of the association. Let us assume we have data from an observational cross-sectional study[12] performed in Italy that show a strong association between duration of direct sun exposure and skin cancer. New data become available from a second cross-sectional study, this time from Spain, also showing a strong association. According to the *proper membership* requirement of Ex-J, we are justified to believe the Spanish data if it is a proper member of the explanatory system *E*, which, until now, consists only of the Italian data. The strong association of the data from Spain are in accord with Hill's viewpoint #1 (*strength*). However, before we can make the Spanish data a component of *E*, we need to also fulfill the second requirement for Ex-J, *superior virtuosity*, which requires that *E* is more virtuous than any alternative explanation *E'*. It is easy to see that this requirement is fulfilled as well, because the Spanish data provide similar evidence from a different population, which satisfies Hill's viewpoint #2, *consistency*. Thus, not only are the Spanish data coherent with the Italian data (which actually satisfies another one of Hill's viewpoints, #7), but also the Spanish and Italian data form a coherent *explanatory system*. If we accept fulfillment of an increasing number of Hill's heuristics as a measure of increasing virtuosity, we are now justified to believe the Spanish data, because they are now a member of E (with Italian and Spanish data as members), which is more virtuous than E' (with only the Italian data).

Let us further assume that new evidence becomes available, this time from a cohort study from Greece that yields a similarly strong measure of association. This third piece of evidence not only satisfies Hill's viewpoints #1, #2, and #7, but also #4, *temporality*.[13] Again, we are justified to believe in the Greek data, because they are now a member of E (*together* with Italian and Spanish data), which is more virtuous than E' (with *only* the Italian and Spanish data), and much more virtuous than E'' (with Italian data only).[14]

8.3.4 Outlook

The earlier designation of Hill's list of viewpoints as explanatory virtues in a coherentist explanatory framework should be considered only the beginning of a broader project. Such a project would need to drill down to what the individual viewpoints #1–#9 exactly entail in light of what others have written. It should also offer comprehensive examples of how the Hill-Poston version of etiological coherentism can be implemented in real-life health science.[15] Moreover, in the remainder of this section, allusion is made to three interesting topics that should be integrated in such future work, that is, a rebuttal of Poston's *primitiveness claim*, a comparative exhibition of etiological coherence theory *versus* unificationist approaches, and a discussion of whether etiological explanations based on the Hill-Poston model fit Claveau's idea of error-independent evidence (Claveau 2012).

8.3.4.1 Epistemic primitivity of explanation à la Poston

Poston considers explanation primitive, that is, he thinks that explanation cannot be analyzed in terms of sufficient and necessary conditions. He starts from the position that explanations remove a mystery, and in science, they often do so by providing a reason why things happen. In parallel to Williamson's argument "that knowledge lacks an analysis into informative necessary and sufficient conditions,"[16] Poston arrives at the conclusion that "we can identify criteria for weighing different explanations, but explanation lacks an informative analysis in terms of necessary and sufficient conditions" (Poston 2014:73). He calls this the *primitiveness claim* and presents three arguments that the nature of explanation is primitive. First, he argues that early in cognitive development, humans start to ask "why" and take "because" for an answer, simply because that is what explanations are supposed to do. He thinks that the ability to appreciate the difference between how things appear and how things are is a quintessential feature of human cognition, and that explanations provide the means to make that differentiation. Poston argues that this capability is so deeply engrained in our human cognitive repertoire that it should be considered fundamental.

Second, he shows that some mathematical proofs are explanatorily different from others. He gives examples of brute force and reduction proofs, which show *that* a claim is true, and contrasts them with constructive proofs, which explain *why* it is true. One reason for the existence of such explanatory difference is that explanation is fundamental.

Third, Poston argues that explanation is epistemically primitive. As an example, he uses *modus ponens*. He holds that

> [a]t the level of a theory of content, we can specify a true logical principle; for example, every admissible interpretation that assigns both "p" and "$p \rightarrow q$" true must assign "q" true. Yet this true principle does not track a metaphysical principle about human inference. (Poston 2014:80)

This absence is what is to be expected if explanatoriness is indeed epistemically primitive. For the present context, this would mean that the *explanation part* of etiological explanations cannot be analyzed, but different etiological explanations can be compared and weighed, which requires the integration of Hill's viewpoints with Poston's explanatory coherentism. Contrary to Poston, however, while explanation may not be reducible to simple underlying concepts, it is explainable. Such meta-explanation would do exactly this, that is, explain how explanations come about; such meta-explanation is precisely what Hempel and Oppenheim, Salmon, van Fraassen, Kitcher, and other philosophers of explanation offered when they offered theirs (Hempel and Oppenheim 1948; Kitcher 1989; Salmon 1984; Van Fraassen Bas 1980). One such meta-explanation is explanatory unification.

8.3.4.2 Explanatory unification

The Hill-Poston approach to etiological explanation has some striking similarities with *explanatory unification*, spearheaded by Michael Friedman and Philip Kitcher (Friedman 1974; Kitcher 1989).

Friedman's account begins with setting his task as finding an objective explication of what it means for a scientific explanation to produce understanding. He outlines and criticizes three traditional accounts of explanation: (1) the D-N model, in which the description of one phenomenon can explain another only by entailing it; (2) the "familiarity" model, in which unfamiliar phenomena can be explained only by references to familiar ones; and (3) the "intellectual fashion" model, in which the overall status of scientific knowledge of an era defines ideals of intelligibility (phenomena that are self-explanatory), to which explananda can be related. Friedman considers it desirable to "isolate a common, objective sense of explanation which remains constant throughout the history of science" (Friedman 1974:13). He calls for a theory that is sufficiently general, is objective, provides a plausible connection between explanation and understanding, and attempts to isolate a property of scientific explanation that has all three of these characteristics. His proposed theory is conveniently simple and elegant: he proposes that the "essence of scientific explanation [is that it] increases our understanding of the world by reducing the total number of independent phenomena that we have to accept as ultimate or given" (p. 15). Friedman gives further details of this proposal and stresses that

> scientific understanding is a global affair. We don't simply replace one phenomenon with another. We replace one phenomenon with a *more comprehensive* phenomenon,

and thereby effect a reduction in the total number of accepted phenomena. (Friedman 1974:19)

In essence, Friedman proposes that explanations unify multiple phenomena into one. In our context, etiological explanations are various characteristics of the etiological process that collectively explain illness occurrence by unifying them into a *more comprehensive* story about how illness comes about, compared to simpler stories that refer to only the causes or only the pathomechanism, and so forth.

Another unificationist account is Kitcher's, which – in a nutshell – purports that "science supplies us with explanations whose worth cannot be appreciated by considering them one by one but only by seeing how they form part of a systematic picture of the order of nature" (Kitcher 1989:430). Kitcher basically agrees with Friedman's account but suggests that science serves the function to "derive descriptions of many phenomena, using the same patterns of derivation again and again, and, in demonstrating this, it teaches us how to reduces the type of facts we have to accept as ultimate" (p. 432). Future work on etiological explanations may attempt to show that this is, indeed, what etiological explanations can do for the health sciences.

8.3.4.3 Evidential heterogeneity and error independence

One interesting "value added" that comes with Hill's list of viewpoints is their *evidential heterogeneity*. It has been suggested that while some of Hill's viewpoints are compatible with a probabilistic *regularity* view of causality, others seem to be in keeping with a *generative* view of causality (Thygesen, Andersen, and Andersen 2005). Others have suggested that while some viewpoints involve mechanistic considerations, others involve probabilistic considerations (Russo and Williamson 2007b). This evidential heterogeneity of Hill's viewpoints works in our favor because it is likely to generate *error independence* of the individual pieces of evidence provided by the individual p_i. Hill's viewpoints represent an explanatory coherentist system that slowly accumulates evidence over time for etiological explanations until consensus in some pertinent community is reached that action is justified. Claveau writes:

> If one has good reason to believe that one type of evidence is unreliable [...] it is hard to see why our belief in the reliability of the other type should be affected. When an evidential set has this property, we can say that its elements are error independent. (Claveau 2012:811)

Thus, the more p we have in any explanatory system E, the larger their heterogeneity (Claveau prefers evidential *variety*), and the higher the likelihood that they are error independent. Moreover, the more error independent p are in a system, the better that system's stability,[17] and thus, the higher the likelihood that it can compete successfully against alternative explanatory systems.

Hill's heuristics remain a stronghold in epidemiology textbook chapters on causal inference. As mere viewpoints to be considered during a decision-making process, they are not considered hard-and-fast criteria for proof of causation. Discussed in this chapter is my proposal that Hill's main goal is to provide a heuristic to justify health interventions based on etiological explanation of observed associations from epidemiological studies. My suggestion is to interpret Hill's framework of viewpoints as an explanatory coherentist system of statements that can stand alone or serve as one element of larger, multidisciplinary systems of scientific evidence. I think that this view reflects well what is going on in current epidemiology and the other health sciences and that a more elaborate and refined version of this proposal might even prove to be a useful tool in efforts to improve individual and population health.

8.4 CONCLUSION

In this book, an analysis of the terms *etiology* and *etiological explanation* from the epidemiological perspective was offered. My point of departure is the claim by epidemiologists, reflected in textbook introductions, that their goal is to find causes of illness. Although this may certainly be the case, and despite their success in doing so, I think that this is a bit of an understatement. At closer examination, it becomes obvious that what epidemiologists really do is something like *contributing evidence for comprehensive etiological explanations*. A sole focus on causes and causal inference in epidemiology seems to be somewhat beside the point, because there is neither an agreed-upon definition in epidemiology of what a cause is nor a unified method that tells us how to find one. The epidemiological community has attempted to clarify these notions, without much success or even consensus. Instead of causation, my focus is on etiology, and instead of causal inference, my focus is on etiological explanation. In what follows, my discussion, findings, and proposal are summarized (Section 8.4.1) and the chapter concludes by defending my proposal against some "big picture" objections, and by briefly sketching two areas of further study.

8.4.1 Summary of proposal

The term *etiology* is used, in the health sciences, as broadly referring to "the causal history of illness." However, there is no unified definition in the literature as to what exactly such a story entails. Similarly, the terms *cause* and *causation* are used rather loosely, without generally agreed-upon definitions. My goal in this book is to offer an account of *etiology* and to provide an initial outline for a theory of *etiological explanation in epidemiology*. Modern epidemiology has grown out of attempts to use population statistics to improve population health. One main branch of epidemiology, *analytical* or *risk factor epidemiology*, collects information about potential risk factors and information about health outcomes from large groups of individuals and calculates estimates of the association between risk factors and outcomes. The classic view in epidemiology is that in some situations, the leap from association to causation is justified. One framework for such inference includes Hill's heuristics, a set of nine qualitative viewpoints about epidemiological evidence that, taken together, provide such justification. Still, many agree that these heuristics are by no means *criteria* in the sense of being necessary and sufficient for causal inference. Thus, many epidemiologists hesitate to talk about causation,[18] while their explicit textbook goal is to identify causes of illness. The focus should be shifted from causation to etiology, the causal origin of illness. In this term, *causal origin* is equivalent with *natural history*, the overarching sequence of events that precede and play a role in illness occurrence. In particular, etiology is the overarching relationship between candidate causes (risk factors for illness), the pathogenetic mechanism they induce (pathogenesis), and the clinical disease that emerges.

In epidemiology, two classic frameworks for causal inference and analysis are Hill's heuristics and Rothman's sufficient-component cause model, respectively. Hill does not say what causation is but offers help for causal inference. Hill's are nine viewpoints (rooted in Mill's philosophy) that, when sufficiently covered by epidemiological evidence, support a causal interpretation of that evidence. Rothman's model (rooted in Mackie's philosophy) allows for the organization of component causes into sufficient causal constellations and, thereby, says what causation looks like, but it does not offer much help with causal inference. A third approach, the *potential outcomes* approach, holds that causation can be extracted from epidemiological data if they come from randomized or quasi-randomized studies.

My suggestion to move from causal inference to etiological explanation is a direct response to Alex Broadbent's invitation to do just this. In keeping with my interpretation of the term *etiology*, I propose to define an *etiological explanation* as *a plausible description of a process of causes, pathogenetic mechanisms, and other contributors in the presence of which illness occurs more frequently than in their absence*. I also provide circumstances under which an etiological explanation is good (if it is a plausible candidate for being the underpinning for intervention design) and useful (when it actually yields improved population health).

In his book *Philosophy of Epidemiology*, Broadbent discusses stability and good prediction as two candidate characteristics of useful epidemiological data. *Intervention* should be added to the mix in the sense of experimental manipulation, a crucial ingredient in both laboratory and epidemiological experiments (randomized controlled trials). Human intervention adds to the explanatory benefits of randomized experiments, usually attributed to the minimization of bias (including confounding) via randomization and blinding. Explanation by intervention comes with the benefit of delivering evidence of efficacy, suggesting potential effectiveness in real-life situations in medicine and public health, thereby improving upon explanations based on stability and good prediction only.

The proposal by Illari and Russo to look at causation in the sciences from a *pluralist mosaicist* perspective is most welcome in the setting of etiological explanations. Since etiological explanations require at least some causal and some pathogenetic evidence, etiological pluralism would entail pluralism of both causes and causation. Such etiological pluralism has been alluded to by one of the pioneers of causal thinking in the health sciences, Mervyn Susser. The heterogeneity of what Susser called *forms of determination* is discussed, drawing on examples from my own work in developmental neuro-epidemiology.

The Russo–Williamson thesis (RWT) holds that causal claims in the health sciences need to be supported by evidence of difference-making (associations) and evidence of mechanism. Going beyond previous points of criticism, my own discussion of the RWT, developed in collaboration with Alex Fiorentino, results in the proposal to (a) think of difference-making as *exposure-outcome* evidence and

(b) rethink mechanistic evidence in the health sciences to include entity-based, association-based, and activity-based mechanistic evidence. Here, it becomes clear that the difference-making claim of the RWT can be nested in the mechanistic claim in the form of association-based mechanistic evidence. In essence, both exposure-outcome evidence and mechanistic evidence require the observation of differences. In one way or another, evidence of mechanism and evidence of difference-making always coexist in causal explanations, thus rendering the RWT true, but only trivially so. In etiological explanations, causal hypotheses explain observed associations that qualify as exposure-outcome evidence, while finer-grained associations and knowledge of entities ultimately explain a causal hypothesis.

Despite its explanatory advantages, mechanistic explanation of health phenomena might place too much emphasis on entities and activities, their organization, and the changes they produce, and pay too little attention to the fact that all etiology is a *process*. This *process perspective* is of crucial importance in the health sciences, because the sequence in which entities are involved in the activities of a mechanism is of greatest interest for the design of interventions. Autism is traditionally considered an all-or-nothing disorder, a disease state that, once it is there, remains there and does not change. Recent evidence from neonatal epidemiology, neuroscience, and immunology suggests that this might not be the whole story. An example from my own work with Carmina Erdei illustrates that many individuals with autism are born preterm (cause) and appear to exhibit an inflammatory response (pathomechanism) that begins at around birth and continues throughout childhood, which is a process that might be a good target for intervention. Thus, an etiological explanation of autism from the process perspective might rescue autistic children from the traditional assumption of being untreatable. Placing these aspects of autism etiology into the Mackie–Rothman framework of sufficient-component causation, and reinterpreting it as a framework for etiological explanations might be particularly useful.

Etiological explanations should not be restricted to causal and pathogenetic components. In what is called *comprehensive* etiological explanations, the concept of *combined contribution* plays an important role as "comprehensifier." Michael Kelly, Rachel Kelly, and Federica Russo have proposed that finding a way to integrate behavioral, social, and biological mechanisms into what they call *mixed mechanisms* would be finding a way to provide better pathogenetic models. In response to their proposal, (1) the biological and social mechanisms are integrated in illness occurrence models more frequently than they appear to think, (2) what they call *pathogenesis* is actually *etiology*, and (3) what is called the *etiological stance* would entail looking at the combined contribution to illness etiology by different kinds of contributors, such as initiators, modifiers, and mediators, and perhaps even background conditions. *Etiological contributor* is defined as any factor that is part of and plays a functional role in an etiological process. This etiological stance would maximize the number of entities, associations, and activities that may be considered targets for intervention.

Finally, in order to be explanatorily relevant, etiological explanations would benefit from being put together according to the framework of explanatory coherentism. When reading Ted Poston's book *Reason and Explanation*, I was struck by how well my vision of etiological explanations resonates with his explanationist theory of justification (Ex-J), which states that one is justified to believe a claim if and only if the claim is part of a sufficiently virtuous explanatory system that beats competitors. In Ex-J lingo, one is justified to believe in a causal or mechanistic claim about aspects of illness occurrence if and only if such a claim is part of a sufficiently virtuous etiological explanation that beats competitors. Hill's list of viewpoints can be joined with Poston's Ex-J such that they provide an explanatory coherentist grid for etiological explanations. More exploratory work will include, for example, a rebuttal of Poston's primitiveness argument (which states that explanation cannot be further reduced but is a fundamental concept), a discussion of whether etiological explanations qualify as unificationist explanations, and an analysis of evidential variety as an explanatory virtue of Hill's heuristics.

In conclusion, I hope to have offered a broad, rigorous, and comprehensive, albeit not necessarily exhaustive, analysis and discussion in support of the argument that it is possible and perhaps even useful to move from causal inference to etiological explanation in epidemiology (Chapter 3). I have also shown how to do this and have offered one way to fit this move into a coherentist approach to explanation. I have argued that etiological pluralism of causes and of causation (Chapter 4) requires the consideration of different kinds of mechanistic evidence (Chapter 5), that a process perspective will be helpful (Chapter 6) when looking at the combined contribution of etiological factors (Chapter 7), and that explanatory coherentism seems to be a viable framework for comprehensive etiological explanations (Chapter 8). I hope that all this will somehow turn out to be helpful for the generation of better interventions designed to improve population health.

A few issues remain to be addressed. In what follows I, first, explain why and how I think the approach of this book sustains its overarching argument. Second, I outline some "big picture" objections and why I think they do not invalidate my work. Third, I briefly sketch two areas into which the arguments I have developed in this book could be expanded.

8.4.2 Defense against some "big picture" objections

First, a "big picture" critic might reject coherentism *in toto*. This objection holds that coherentist explanations do not work because coherence is not anchored in *anything*. In other words, my proposal to design etiological explanations as explanations of the coherentist kind will fail because coherentism fails. Such an anticoherentist critic would need to offer an alternative to coherentism, for example, some sort of foundationalism, which holds that there *must* be an absolute, irrefutable basis for an explanation to be valid. To my knowledge, however, no such foundationalist view has ever been successfully offered in the philosophy of science. To this, the anticoherentist could argue that she does not need to provide an alternative view, because providing alternative views is not a necessary component of a rejection. My response would be that I would accept the anticoherentist argument if the critic could convince me that the explanatory coherentist view is fatally flawed. In epidemiological practice, the justification of beliefs in details of etiological explanations depends very much on *background knowledge*, which means that most of our beliefs about new data depend on our beliefs in background data. I am not aware of *any* piece of etiological knowledge that goes back to a piece of *a priori* knowledge. However, even if foundationalism were true, this does not necessarily mean that coherentism is wrong. If there is some truth to either one, perhaps hybrid approaches such as Susan Haack's foundherentism and her associated crossword-puzzle analogy might be a good fit for etiological explanations (Haack 1993). Unfortunately, this interesting topic is far beyond the scope of this book and will have to wait for another day.

Second, causal skeptics might argue that *causation has no place in etiological explanations because the very concept of causation is blurred.* This stance goes back to Russell's oft-cited position according to which there are no such things as causes and that, therefore, the concept should be done away with (Russell 1913). Etiological explanations are causal-mechanical explanations. If one doubts the very existence of causes, then one should also doubt the existence of etiology, which would render etiological explanations meaningless. If that were true, the skeptic would need to clarify how medicine and public health could have been as successful as they were over the past centuries if not with the help of causal inference and prediction. That success is just too good to be the result of sheer dumb luck. Another kind of causal skepticism does not reject the idea of causation but only holds that "one may doubt that we have any clear and univocal notion" of causation (Healey 2009). As discussed in Chapter 4, I suggest that etiological pluralism is causal *and* pathogenetic pluralism, which makes it immune to the potential downsides of the absence of such unified notion. In the health sciences, the kinds of etiological stories we tell range from stories about accidents via stories about accidents to stories about tumorigenesis, and to stories about psychodynamics. *Not* having a clear and univocal account of causation might rather be *helpful* with the design of etiological explanations under all these various etiological circumstances.

Third, someone might say that we cannot move from causal inference to etiological explanation because *causal inference and causal explanation are the same.* I disagree, mainly because causal inference is giving an answer to a simple "yes" or "no" question, such as: does excessive sun exposure cause skin cancer? A causal explanation, on the other hand, answers a "why" question by not just stating *that* excessive sun exposure might cause skin cancer, but also by providing information about the causal mechanism of how the sun does this. Etiological explanations are a certain kind of causal explanation, as outlined by Salmon: "Etiological explanations are, of course, thoroughly causal; they explain a given fact by showing how it came to be as a result of antecedent events, processes, and conditions" (Salmon 1984:269). In keeping with this view, I think of causal inference and causal explanation as two very different things.

Fourth, another objection could come from the angle of the *potential outcomes approach* (POE). The POE defender could state that we do not need etiological explanations since we can have suitable causal inference using the POE. My response is to assure that the POE cannot replace etiological explanations because these go beyond causal inference, by integrating causal with mechanistic facts into comprehensive explanations, and by including information about contributors such as mediators, modifiers, and so forth. From this perspective, it may well be fruitful to consider integrating the POA as one technique to generate data for etiological explanations (see later), but not to replace it with the POA, because at least part of the story will be lost. For the same reason, another POA defender could say that while both the Hill heuristics and the POA are valid and have their place in epidemiology, the POA is the more recent (modern) approach and Hill's approach is outdated (classic). This is exactly the view put forward by Glass and coauthors (Glass et al. 2013) but without supporting evidence that justifies the conclusion that it is invalid or even just less effective than the POA, just because it is the older concept. The POA builds on work by Donald Rubin that dates back to the early 1970s, less than a decade after Hill published his seminal paper, so it is not much more recent (Hill 1965; Rubin 1974). As an aside, the main concept behind the POA, the generation of quasi-randomized data from observational studies for the purpose of causal inference, was considered by the same Sir Austin Bradford Hill much earlier (in 1953) when he asked, "can observations be made in such a way as to fulfill, as far as possible, experimental requirements?" (Hill 1953:995). Experiment is also one of the nine Hill viewpoints, and nothing in Hill's paper indicates that he was referring to laboratory experiments exclusively. Thus, one important, if not the most important foundation of the POA was considered essential for causal inference almost two decades before the POA was born.

What's next? In fact, to *integrate etiological explanations with the POA* would be one interesting way to move forward. I have not discussed the POA in detail in this book, because it deals mainly with causal inference, which I suggest leaving behind (or at least put aside for a while). Others have recently offered a cogent critique elsewhere.[19] What might be worthwhile would be an attempt to bring quantitative aspects from the POA into the predominantly qualitative way of constructing etiological explanations. As mentioned earlier, Hill has *experiment* as one of his viewpoints. This clearly refers back to the idea that a randomized study design carries epistemic value when it comes to causal inference. I have begun, with Ryan Flanagan, to explore this idea of epistemological weight of randomized trials as consisting of epistemological value (methodological quality), function (relationship to other kinds of evidence), and utility (extrapolation of results, increased understanding, clinical usefulness) (Flanagan and Dammann 2018). In this scenario, some concepts from POE might come in handy as a tool to establish epistemological value.

Another interesting topic to explore will be to see whether a coherentist framework can not only be applied to etiological explanations in epidemiology but also to the prediction of interventional success in population health. If a collection of error-independent pieces of evidence arranged as a series of coherent responses to Hill's checkpoints can provide a comprehensive etiological explanation, could a collection of error-independent predictions about interventional success provide a justification for such intervention at the population level? In other words, can one conceive of *predictive coherence* as the basis for the justification of action in population health? This brings up multiple interesting questions. One is the question of how explanation and prediction are related. Hempel, for example, held that explanations, predictions, and post-dictions share the same logical structure (his *symmetry thesis*), an argument that does not stand unchallenged (Fetzer 2017). Another question is whether good explanations are necessarily a good basis for good predictions. If so, what exactly is it that makes good explanations a basis for good predictions, and what is the reason that some predictions fail even if they are based on good predictions?[20] A third question would be what makes a prediction good. Not much has been written about prediction in philosophy of science, so a lot remains to be explored.

Both of these possibilities, exploring the integration of the POE and predictive coherentism in population health, would be attractive topics for future research. At the time of this writing, I tend toward the second, predictive coherentism, as the topic of my next project in philosophy of epidemiology. I look forward to many interesting discussions with my colleagues at the interdisciplinary intersection of philosophy and epidemiology.

ENDNOTES

CHAPTER 1

1. Storrs, C. Kid couch potatoes court long-term health risk. CNN health. Retrieved from http://www.cnn.com/2015/09/30/health/sitting-kids-heart-health/index.html (accessed January 10, 2015).
2. This is sometimes called the "missing data problem," a misnomer in my mind, because the information is not missing but is impossible to obtain – one just *cannot* take *and* not take a pill and, thus, the actual outcome in both situations cannot be compared.
3. I sometimes refer to these two levels of explanation as *macro-* and *micro-etiological levels*, respectively.
4. For details, see Sections 2.5.2.1 and 2.4.1, respectively.

CHAPTER 2

1. In this book, I refer to risk factors as candidate causes. This is what some have called "determinants" of illness occurrence (Susser 1973:3). Susser defines a determinant as "any factor, whether event, characteristic, or other definable entity, so long as it brings about change for better or worse in a health condition." I avoid this term because of the circularity of this definition, due to the similar meaning of the verbs "to determine" and "to bring about."
2. Morabia suggests that group comparisons are the very core of epidemiological thinking (Morabia 2014).
3. See Section 2.5.2.1 and Chapter 8 for more on Hill's viewpoints.
4. Comprehensive textbooks about the theoretical underpinnings and inferential fine points of epidemiology include *Theoretical Epidemiology* (Miettinen 1985), *Modern Epidemiology* (Rothman 1986; Rothman, Greenland, and Lash 2008b), and *Interpreting Epidemiological Evidence* (Savitz 2003).
5. See Chapter 6 for a detailed discussion of the process perspective of etiology.
6. I perceive a direct line of thought here, coming from J. S. Mill (1806–1873) to Mackie (1917–1981) to Rothman. In the 1970s, it was textbook knowledge that "just as any effect has multiple causes, the alteration of any cause may be expected to have multiple effects besides the one intended" (MacMahon and Pugh 1970:26). This view stands in stark contrast to the Henle-Koch postulates; see Chapter 2 in Evans (1993).

7. Throughout this book, I use the term *mechanism* to refer to the biological pathogenetic process that connects exposure and outcome, without commitment to any of the definitions of and discussions about mechanisms in the recent philosophical literature (Bechtel 2011; Broadbent 2011; Clarke et al. 2013b; Craver and Darden 2013; Glennan 1996; Glennan 2008; Illari and Williamson 2012; Machamer, Darden, and Craver 2000).

8. This is outlined in more detail in Chapter 7.

9. I deliberately refrain from offering a historical survey here. Those interested may want to read Alfred Evans (1993) and Kay Codell Carter (2003).

10. See, *inter alia*, Dawid (2004); Dekkers and Rikkert (2006); Doll (2002); Evans (1978); Flier and de Vries Robbé (1999); Greenland and Brumback (2002); Greenland (1999); Hernán (2004); Hernan and Robins (2006a); Hill (1965); Krieger (1994); Lilienfeld (1959); Little and Rubin (2000); Maldonado and Greenland (2002); Parascandola and Weed (2001); Pearce (1990); Petersen, Sinisi, and van der Laan (2006); Philippe and Mansi (1998); Räisänen et al. (2006); Renton (1994); Rizzi (1994); Rizzi and Pedersen (1992); Robins (2001); Rothman (1976); Rubin (1997); Samuels (1998); Sartwell (1960); Scheutz and Poulsen (1999); Susser (1977, 1991); Weed (1986); Weed (2008); and Yerushalmy and Palmer (1959).

11. See Beebee, Hitchcock, and Menzies (2009) for a comprehensive overview.

12. See Section 2.4.1 for a more detailed description of this model.

13. This definition underlies the potential outcomes approach (POA) referred to in Section 2.5.2.2.

14. Ibid.

15. See Rothman (1976). In the epidemiological literature, this model is called the *sufficient-component cause model*.

16. The necessary piece (A) in the sufficient-component framework appears to be modeled after Mackie's INUS condition (Mackie 1965, 1974).

17. See Chapter 7 for more on contribution.

18. See later in this chapter and Section 6.2.

19. See, for example, Mill (1856: chapter V).

20. This concept has, to my knowledge, been revisited (Rothman, Greenland, and Lash 2008b) but not modified (see, later, my suggested modification that includes the time arrow and makes all this a process). Aspects of it had previously been discussed by Susser (1973), who later (1991) traced the concept of necessary and sufficient causes back to Galileo, via Bunge, who quotes Il Saggiatore (1623), (Bunge 1979).

21. Unpublished manuscript, 1994.

22. For details on induction time and latent periods see Rothman (1981).

23. In Figure 2.3, all component causes have their onset and offset at the same time. This is for ease of depiction only – in actual illness causation, both onset and offset of causal factors are likely to occur at multiple different time points.

24. For the sake of brevity, I refer in what follows to only two brief pieces describing Mumford and Anjum's account of dispositionalist causation, the first chapter in Mumford and Anjum (2011a) and a paper published in the clinical care literature that relates to their account (Kerry et al. 2012).

25. It also fits John Dupré's notion of biological processes (Dupré 2013). This account deemphasizes the recent focus on mechanisms in biology, see, for example, Nicholson (2012), and champions a process view of biological causation that goes well beyond physical accounts of process causation; see Dowe (2000), Dowe (2009), and Salmon (1984, 1998).

26. RR = Risk for outcome given exposure/Risk for outcome in the absence of exposure.

27. Vandenbroucke (1998).

28. Fagot-Largeault (1989). I am grateful to Jan Vandenbroucke for bringing this reference and his referring article to my attention.

29. Vandenbroucke (1998:SII 16). With "hypothetic-deductive," Vandenbroucke refers to scientific methods rooted in Popperian falsificationist reasoning. Between 1975 and the late 1990s, Popper's philosophy was a hot topic in the epidemiological literature (see, for example, Buck 1975, 1989; Greenland 1988, 1998; Jacobsen 1976; Karhausen 1995; Maclure 1985; Pearce and Crawford-Brown 1989; Susser 1986; Weed 1985, 1988). A full discussion of this debate has to wait for another day.

30. Hippocrates. *On Airs, Waters, and Places* (translated by Francis Adams). Retrieved from http://classics.mit.edu/Hippocrates/airwatpl.html (accessed January 16, 2019).

31. Using similar reasoning, Gary Taubes, at the time editor of the highly respected journal *Science,* lamented a lack of certainty in risk factor epidemiology in a somewhat polemic but interesting article that captures the tension between epidemiology, the press, and the public created by difficulties distinguishing between correlation and causation (Taubes 1995).

32. See also Dammann and Leviton (2007).

33. As Ludwik Fleck wrote in 1935: "The individual is the soccer player, the thought collective is the team, and the game is the epistemic process" (Fleck 1935 [2012]:62), translation mine.

34. Hernan, M. *Causal Inference: What If.* Boca Raton, FL: Chapman & Hall/ CRC. Retrieved from http://www.hsph.harvard.edu/miguel-hernan/causal-inference-book/ (accessed November 2, 2015).

35. See Susser (2004) and Susser and Susser (1996) for an epidemiological perspective on levels of causation.

36. See Glass et al. (2013), Hernán (2004), Hernan and Robins (2006a), Parascandola and Weed (2001), Rothman (1976), Susser (1973), Susser (1991), Weed (1986), and Weed (2008) for an overview.

37. See Hill (1965), Phillips and Goodman (2006), Rothman and Greenland (1998), Susser (1977), Ward (2009a,b), and Weed (1988).

38. See, for example, Savitz (2003) and Weed (2008).

39. See Weed (2008:footnote 14).

40. Weed (2008). In a footnote, Weed adds that "it is reasonable to assume that some scientists' judgments are better than others." How can that be, however, if any judgment about causation would need to be judged against a solid reference frame as well?

41. See Doll (2002) for an interesting perspective on deduction of causality from epidemiological observation that, surprisingly, has the word *proof* in its title.

42. See, for example, Höfler (2005, 2006), Lucas and McMichael (2005), Morabia (2013), Phillips and Goodman (2004, 2006), Poole (2001), Ward (2009a,b), Weed (1997), and Worrall (2011).
43. See Glass et al. (2013) and Section 2.5.2.2.
44. See Chapter 8.
45. For example, those by Anders Ahlbom and Staffan Norell, pages 93–8 and 129–35 in Nordenfelt and Lindahl (1984), respectively.
46. As far as I know, Ahlbom and Norell are epidemiologists, not philosophers.
47. Ibid., 257.
48. Ibid., 271.
49. Dawid, Faigman, and Fienberg (2014:360).
50. Ibid.
51. Dawid, Faigman, and Fienberg (2014:383).
52. Ibid.
53. Rose (1985).
54. Wetzel (2018). Retrieved from https://plato.stanford.edu/archives/fall2018/entries/types-tokens/ (accessed April 2, 2019).
55. Peirce (1906:505–6).
56. *Outbreaks* are epidemics in defined geographical areas. *Epidemic* is defined as disease occurrence at an incidence rate that is clearly exceeding expected levels in a particular time frame in a particular population. See Oleckno (2008).
57. Centers for Disease Control and Prevention. Measles cases in 2019. Retrieved from https://www.cdc.gov/measles/cases-outbreaks.html (accessed April 2, 2019).
58. See Mumford and Anjum (2011a:107).
59. I will not address the possibility of "backward causation," a.k.a., "retro-causation"; see Faye (2018).
60. Gelman calls this "forward" and "reverse causal inference"; see Gelman (2011).
61. On his McGill University website, Miettinen lists as his area of expertise "theory of medicine and public health and of medical research, epidemiologic and meta-epidemiologic, forming the knowledge base of scientific medicine."
62. Miettinen and Karp (2012:36).
63. Ibid.
64. Ibid.; emphasis mine.
65. *Incidence* is the number of new cases in a time unit per all individuals at risk at the beginning of that time unit.
66. *Prevalence* is the number of individuals with a certain health condition or disease per all individuals in a population, at a certain time point or over a certain stretch of time.
67. Miettinen and Karp distinguish between "etiology as a community-medicine concern" and "etiology as a clinical medicine concern," but their emphasis is on the respective roles these concepts play in community-level and patient-level intervention planning, not on how they differ metaphysically and epistemically (Miettinen and Karp 2012:38–40).
68. The idea of causal vigor needs further development. For the time being, I consider it to be the causal equivalent (if there is such a thing) of "strength of association," as, for example, in Hill (1965).
69. Dawid, Faigman, and Fienberg (2014:375).

CHAPTER 3

1. Of course, in order to explain this *cogently*, the common cause scenario must be more plausible than the putative causal exposure scenario.
2. Ibid., p. 905. Finding the *best* definition requires comparison to alternatives, which is a critical feature of inference to the best explanation and of explanatory coherentism (see Chapter 8 of this book).
3. Chapter 7 provides a detailed discussion of my framework of *etiological explanation*.
4. See, for example, Gordis (2014:2), Oleckno (2008:1), and Webb and Bain (2011:17).
5. See earlier in this chapter, Section 2.5.2.2, and Glass et al. (2013), Hernán (2004), Hernán and Robins (2006b), Imbens and Rubin (2015), and VanderWeele (2015).
6. See, for example, Rubin (1974).
7. See, for example, Pearl (1988).
8. Perhaps this is with the exception of molecular and genetic epidemiological studies, which often include biomarkers for mechanistic processes.
9. This point has been offered to me by Alex Broadbent.
10. See Chapter 7 for a more detailed discussion of micro- and macro-etiology.
11. Note that this account of causality in the health sciences is different from that proposed by Russo and Williamson (2007b), although the accounts may look almost identical. While Russo and Williamson think we need evidence of both difference-making and mechanism, I suggest that we need both macrolevel and microlevel etiological evidence, and that difference-making and mechanistic aspects play a role at both levels. I have started working on this proposal with Alex Fiorentino (Fiorentino and Dammann 2015), but a comprehensive discussion has to wait for another day.
12. In some cases, epidemiological research can help mount the evidence in support of both causal and causal-mechanical explanation. Molecular epidemiology is usually seen as being capable of going beyond mere exposure-outcome relationships by shedding some light on the molecular mechanisms at work between exposure and outcome; see Schulte and Perera (1993).
13. This macro-etiological evidence is what Alex Fiorentino and I have come to call *exposure-outcome evidence*; see Fiorentino and Dammann (2015).
14. See, for example, Dammann and Leviton (1997, 2004).
15. Fleck 1935 (2012) (translation from German mine).
16. This is not to be confused with evidence needed to justify public health intervention. Smoking cessation programs are fully justified despite the glaring lack of knowledge about a causal mechanism.
17. One has to be mindful that in order to justify activities targeted at the design of medical or public health interventions, GEEs are sufficient. Strictly speaking, the label *UEE* can be given only to explanations that have stood the test of time.
18. Useful etiological explanations as defined earlier will be *particularly* useful if they help achieve the goals of public health and medicine. This notion resonates with Woodward, who takes usefulness to be "the only standard that

matters" when he describes what he calls his "functional project" as the "idea that causal information and reasoning are sometimes useful or functional in the sense of serving various goals and purposes" (Woodward 2014).

19. See, for example, Rubin (2007).

20. One particularly interesting facet of the RCT concept worthy of discussion is the epistemological status of computer simulations of RCTs. Unfortunately, this goes far beyond the scope of this book.

21. Of course, there are many other limitations of the manipulationist approach in the health sciences. For example, no one would seriously suggest using manipulation to study adverse health effects of, say, smoking or asbestos without violating ethical boundaries.

22. I use "observational studies" in quotation marks as synonymous with noninterventional epidemiological studies such as cohort, case-control, and cross-sectional studies.

23. In Sections 2.5.2.1 and 2.5.2.2, respectively.

24. For a more detailed discussion, see Chapter 8.

25. See, for example, VanderWeele (2015:4–5).

26. Some early pioneers of evidence-based medicine went as far as suggesting ignoring observational data if data from randomized trials are available.

27. With Ryan Flanagan, I have started developing this theme toward the idea that the epistemological weight of RCTs depends on their results (see Flanagan and Dammann 2018).

28. Some would call this evidence of difference-making. In RCTs, this difference is mainly due to modification by the drug of a pathogenetic pathway.

29. This is why some have come to use the term *effect-measure modification* (Rothman and Mahon 2004).

30. The arguably "classic" debate about this issue was initiated by Howson and Urbach (1993), Urbach (1993), and Worrall (2007), who cogently criticized the perceived epistemological superiority of RCTs. Among the defenders of RCTs are Papineau (1994) and La Caze (2013).

31. But not usually to the elucidation of pathogenetic mechanisms, which is the turf of the laboratory sciences. Molecular and genetic epidemiological studies might be exceptions.

32. It needs to be further explored whether the suggestion to transition from causal inference to causal explanation (Broadbent 2013) can and/or should be integrated that causal claims in the biomedical sciences need support from both mechanistic and difference-making evidence (Russo and Williamson 2007b).

33. Thanks to Alex Broadbent for bringing this point to my attention.

34. Per Broadbent's framework, RCTs also need to be stable and yield good predictions to be able to offer this kind of information. Thus, ideally, multiple clinical trials are needed to arrive at a solid causal explanation from RCTs.

35. This line of reasoning has come to be called the "Russo–Williamson thesis" (Russo and Williamson 2007b). Briefly, it states that causal claims in the health sciences need to gather support from both difference-making and mechanistic evidence. For a comprehensive discussion, see Chapter 5.

CHAPTER 4

1. Illari and Russo use the "mosaic" metaphor for their proposed causal pluralist perspective (see later and Chapter 23 of *Causality: Philosophical Theory Meets Scientific Practice*).
2. See Rothman (1976) and Section 2.4.1.
3. Craver was not the first to use the "mosaic" metaphor (Charlton 1996; Lewis 1986:ix).
4. If this is indeed what those who do exposomics research think they do, the term *exposomics* is a misnomer and should be replaced with the term *exposology*. If instead exposomics is what the term denotes, it is the idea to consider *all* lifetime exposures and their individual and joint health effects. (See Coughlin, 2014, for a concise discussion of exposomics in light of multiple other -omics approaches.)
5. See, for example, Figure 1.2 in Schulte and Perera (1993:6).
6. Or at least, as they say in parts of the United States, "'til the cows come home."
7. Godfrey-Smith laments that many do not explicitly distinguish between these two kinds of pluralism (Godfrey-Smith 2009:327–8).
8. He calls the other two kinds of pluralism noted earlier, *metaphysical* and *conceptual* pluralism, respectively.
9. For a comprehensive defense of evidential pluralism in epidemiology, see Broadbent, Vandenbroucke, and Pearce (2016) and Vandenbroucke, Broadbent, and Pearce (2016).
10. In Dammann (2017) and in Chapter 7 of this book.
11. Mayo Clinic. Cancer. Retrieved from https://www.mayoclinic.org/diseases-conditions/cancer/symptoms-causes/syc-20370588
12. Those later causes of gene mutations (smoking, radiation, and viruses, among many others) are also plural in two ways: (1) in what they are and (2) in how they come about. With regard to (1), smoke is a cloud of particulate matter in air resulting from tobacco combustion, radiation is energy (or particles) moving through space (or matter) in waveform, and viruses are clumps of genetic code wrapped in protein. With regard to (2), exposure to tobacco smoke is mainly the result of a behavior, radiation can come from either natural (sun) or nonnatural sources (tanning beds), and both kinds of exposure can often be modified by choice; viruses are ubiquitous in the human environment and are transferred in multiple ways between organisms.
13. This is how we distinguish different kinds of prevention: primary (eliminate illness), secondary (ameliorate illness), and tertiary (prevent consequences of illness). Not coincidentally, these activities define different kinds of health care as performed in public health, medicine, and rehabilitation, respectively.
14. Later in this book, the same concept is applied to the etiology of autism (in Chapter 6). My version of what Susser called *multiple causality* is also developed, called *combined contribution* (in Chapter 7).
15. See Section 2.4.1. It is also reflected in my discussion of *combined contributions* discussed in Chapter 7.

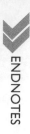

16. See Susser (1973:68). This causal dyad, early brain damage and subsequent development, has been proposed and discussed by Malaeb and Dammann (2009) and by Volpe (2009) as *two separate* causal factors in neurodevelopmental disability.

CHAPTER 5

1. For example, Broadbent (2011), Claveau (2012), Gillies (2011), and Illari (2011).
2. F. Russo, personal communication, November 27, 2015.
3. See, for example, Broadbent (2011), Claveau (2012), Fiorentino and Dammann (2015), Gillies (2011), Illari (2011), and Joffe (2013).
4. See Chapter 9 in Williamson (2005) and Williamson (2006).
5. I have yet to identify the point in either author's writings that tells us in a straightforward manner how to distinguish between causal and noncausal associations based on data alone.
6. Oxford Learner's Dictionaries. Retrieved from http://www.oxfordlearners dictionaries.com/us/definition/english/account-for; accessed July 22, 2016.
7. See, for example, Giere (1997)
8. See Section 2.5.2.2 for a brief introduction to the concept.
9. Ignaz Semmelweis (1818–1865) was a Hungarian physician who introduced antiseptic handwashing to prevent puerperal fever without any knowledge about the disease mechanism. See Csoka (2016) for an interesting discussion of the fact that Semmelweis was ridiculed for his helpful idea, while a generation later, Egas Moniz (1874–1955) received the Nobel prize for introducing lobotomy, which in some cases turned out to be harmful rather than helpful (Lerner 2005).
10. Although some appear to think that a pathomechanism is not really a mechanism, but an irregularity of normal body function (Garson 2013).
11. This view is expanded in Chapter 8 of this book, which deals with coherence in etiological explanations.

CHAPTER 6

1. While the etiology of most diseases may be explained by an outline of the biological process, at least some might be better explained by a more inclusive approach, such as the biopsychosocial model of disease (see Engel 1980; Fava and Sonino 2008).
2. See Figures 4.1 and 7.1.
3. In the spirit of full disclosure, I should mention that I am currently a member of the editorial board of that journal.
4. This section builds on a previous publication (Erdei and Dammann 2014). I am grateful to Carmina Erdei for her permission to use this coauthored material here.

5. See Bechtel (2008, 2011); Craver (2007); Garson (2013); Glennan (2002); Machamer, Darden, and Craver (2000); and Williamson (2011a,b). Two sub-foci of this discourse are directly relevant to biomedicine, i.e., the role of mechanisms in biology (Bechtel 2011; Chao 2013; Nicholson 2012) and in epidemiology (Broadbent 2011; Clarke et al. 2013a,b; Fiorentino and Dammann 2015; Kincaid 2011; Russo 2009; Severinsen 2001).

6. See Section 7.3 for a discussion of contributors to the etiological process.

7. An interesting overview of DNA methylation can be found in Schubeler (2015).

8. The mammalian target of rapamycin pathway is a crucial component of cell growth regulation.

9. See Kleinberg and Hripcsak (2011) on biomedical informatics, Braunstein and Ingrosso (2016) on computational epidemiology, and Mercuri and Baigrie (2016) on medical malpractice litigation.

10. Consider, for example this explanation for the lay audience: "Exposure to UV radiation is the main factor that causes skin cells to become cancer cells. Almost all skin cancers (approximately 99% of non-melanoma skin cancers and 95% of melanoma) are caused by too much UV radiation from the sun or other sources" (Cancer Council NSW. How ultraviolet (UV) radiation causes skin cancer. Retrieved from http://www.cancercouncil.com.au/63295/cancer-prevention/sun-protection/sun-protection-sport-and-recreation/sun-protection-information-for-sporting-groups/how-ultraviolet-uv-radiation-causes-skin-cancer/; accessed May 8, 2016.)

11. "UV radiation is made up of UVA and UVB rays which are able to penetrate the skin and cause permanent damage to the cells below [...] If the body is unable to repair this damage the cell can begin to divide and grow in an uncontrolled way. This growth can eventually form a tumour" (ibid.).

12. Phil Dowe summarized his view in a personal communication thus: "A process is an actual concrete thing, whereas a mechanism is a system of actual and possible processes" (email, January 26, 2015). This driver driving this car to work today is the concrete thing (process), and the driver and car together represent the system of actual or possible drivings (mechanism).

13. Rube Goldberg machines are a good example, e.g., https://www.youtube.com/watch?v=qybUFnY7Y8w

14. Gene Ontology Consortium. Gene ontology overview. Retrieved from http://geneontology.org/page/biological-process-ontology-guidelines

15. Gene Ontology Consortium. Gene ontology overview. Retrieved from http://geneontology.org/page/ontology-documentation

16. Aronson refers to Collingwood (1972) and Gasking (1955).

17. See Section 4.4.3 for a discussion of causes versus conditions.

CHAPTER 7

1. What they probably mean is association, not correlation.

2. This is obviously a change in name only, not in meaning. At most, it is a restriction of meaning to epidemiological contexts.

3. See Vinten-Johansen (2003) for a comprehensive and well-researched biography of John Snow.

4. See, for example, Emmert-Streib and Dehmer (2010).

5. "If E_1 is the cause of E_2, then a small variation (a mark) in E_1 is associated with a small variation in E_2, whereas small variations in E_2 are not associated with variations in E_1," (italics in original).

6. The quote is from Mill's *System of Logic*, Book III, Chapter 5, Section 3, as quoted by Mackie (1974).

7. A "taxonomy of causal explanations" as suggested by Räisänen et al. might be a helpful step in this direction (Räisänen et al. 2006).

8. In some areas of health care, especially in efforts to improve patient safety, the idea of a "root-cause analysis" is that rigorous analysis of adverse event scenarios in health-care settings such as hospitals may help prevent such unforeseen incidents (Vincent 2003). Although this seems to be a perfectly reasonable and laudable attempt to improve health care, it has been emphasized that "root-cause analysis" is a misnomer, because it oversimplifies the idea of causation in health care by reducing it to the idea that adverse events have single causes, and because analyses that focus on incidents are likely to ignore the big picture, the insufficiencies of the "system" that have given rise to the error that led to the event (Vincent 2004).

9. In philosophy, causal power theories capture this phenomenon rather well. See, for example, Cartwright (1989), Mumford (2009), and Mumford and Anjum (2011a).

10. Figure 7.4 is based on Figure 2.3.1 in Woodward (2003:49).

11. Woodward adds that "[d]irect causes will thus always be contributing causes, but there may be contributing causes that are not direct" (Woodward 2003:50).

12. Mediator analysis is an important component of epidemiological data analysis. See, for example, Richiardi, Bellocco, and Zugna (2013) and VanderWeele (2015). Unfortunately, even a brief discussion of its intricacies is far beyond the scope of this book.

CHAPTER 8

1. See pages iv–v in Ross (1965).

2. Quoted verbatim from Thagard (2006).

3. This section is based on a manuscript that has in the meantime evolved into a chapter coauthored with Paul Thagard and Ted Poston; see Dammann, Poston, and Thagard (2019). The section is, however, authored solely by myself and thus reflects my thoughts, not theirs.

4. See Section 2.5.2.1 for a brief overview.

5. See earlier, aspect 7 in list in Section 2.5.2.1.

6. Thanks to Alex Broadbent for pointing this out to me.

7. See Deemter (2010) for a popular account of inexactitude subtitled "in praise of vagueness."

8. This notion resonates with Cartwright's focus on *usage* in causal inference; see Cartwright (2007).

9. From this angle, Hill's proposal looks like a response given half a century before Broadbent made his recent suggestion that "causation and causal inference are overemphasized in epidemiology and epidemiological methodology, and explanation and prediction deserve greater emphasis" (Broadbent 2013:8).

10. This is Broadbent's wording, not mine.

11. All nine of Hill's viewpoints are listed in Section 2.5.2.1.

12. Cross-sectional studies collect information about exposure (sun) and outcome (skin cancer) at the same time; there is no time lag in between the two information collection exercises.

13. Cohort studies assess exposure first, then wait for longer periods of time (years) for the outcome to develop. Thus, the cohort study asserts that the sun exposure came before the skin cancer, hence fulfilling Hill's viewpoint #4 (*temporality*), while the cross-sectional studies cannot.

14. There may certainly be further criteria that help decide whether E or E' wins the competition. A complete discussion of such possibility is far beyond the scope of this book.

15. For one example, see Dammann, Poston, and Thagard (2019).

16. Poston (2014:72), citing Williamson (2000).

17. By referring to stability here, I am tipping my hat to Alex Broadbent's discussion of stability as one central requirement for epidemiological results in order to justify their application in decisions about population health interventions; see Broadbent (2013:59–65) and all of his Chapter 5.

18. The *American Journal of Public Health* has a section of articles on the C-Word in their May 2018 issue. Several authors get very serious about the question of whether or not to articulate causal claims in their work. Part of my motivation for this book is my position that such discussions are slightly beside the point, because a narrow focus on causal inference is, I think, less helpful than a broader one, on etiological explanation.

19. See Broadbent, Vandenbroucke, and Pearce (2016) and Vandenbroucke, Broadbent, and Pearce (2016).

20. Some power theorists of causation suggest that power-based predictions can fail due to the influence of extra powers (Mumford and Anjum 2011a).

REFERENCES

Aden, U., G. Favrais, F. Plaisant, M. Winerdal, U. Felderhoff-Mueser, J. Lampa, V. Lelievre, and P. Gressens. 2010. Systemic inflammation sensitizes the neonatal brain to excitotoxicity through a pro-/anti-inflammatory imbalance: Key role of TNFα pathway and protection by etanercept. *Brain Behav Immun* 24 (5):747–58.

Ahlbom, A. 1984. Criteria of causal association in epidemiology. In *Health, Disease, and Causal Explanations in Medicine*, edited by L. Nordenfelt and B. I. B. Lindahl, 93–8. Dordrecht, Netherlands: D. Reidel Publishing.

Alvarado, S. G., K. Lenkov, B. Williams, and R. D. Fernald. 2015. Social crowding during development causes changes in GnRH1 DNA methylation. *PLOS ONE* 10 (10):e0142043.

Anscombe, G. E. M. 1993. Causality and determination. In *Causation*, edited by E. Sosa and M. Tooley, 88–104. Oxford, UK: Oxford University Press.

Anthonisen, N. R., M. A. Skeans, R. A. Wise, J. Manfreda, R. E. Kanner, J. E. Connett, and Group Lung Health Study Research. 2005. The effects of a smoking cessation intervention on 14.5-year mortality: A randomized clinical trial. *Ann Intern Med* 142 (4):233–9.

Aronson, J. L. 1971. On the grammar of "cause." *Synthese* 22:414–30.

Ashwood, P., P. Krakowiak, I. Hertz-Picciotto, R. Hansen, I. Pessah, and J. Van de Water. 2011. Elevated plasma cytokines in autism spectrum disorders provide evidence of immune dysfunction and are associated with impaired behavioral outcome. *Brain Behav Immun* 25 (1):40–5.

Atladottir, H. O., T. B. Henriksen, D. E. Schendel, and E. T. Parner. 2012. Autism after infection, febrile episodes, and antibiotic use during pregnancy: An exploratory study. *Pediatrics* 130 (6):e1447–54.

Bakare, M. O., A. O. Agomoh, P. O. Ebigbo, J. Eaton, K. O. Okonkwo, J. U. Onwukwe, and G. M. Onyeama. 2009. Etiological explanation, treatability and preventability of childhood autism: A survey of Nigerian healthcare workers' opinion. *Ann Gen Psychiatry* 8:6.

Banker, B. Q. and J. C. Larroche. 1962. Periventricular leukomalacia of infancy. *Arch Neurol* 7:386–410.

Barros, D. B. 2013. Negative causation in causal and mechanistic explanation. *Synthese* 190 (3):449–69.

Barttfeld, P., B. Wicker, S. Cukier, S. Navarta, S. Lew, and M. Sigman. 2011. A big-world network in ASD: Dynamical connectivity analysis reflects a deficit in long-range connections and an excess of short-range connections. *Neuropsychologia* 49 (2):254–63.

Bechtel, W. 2008. *Mental Mechanisms: Philosophical Perspectives on Cognitive Neuroscience.* New York, NY: Routledge.

Bechtel, W. 2011. Mechanism and biological explanation. *Philos Sci* 78:533–57.

Bechtel, W. and A. Abrahamsen. 2005. Explanation: A mechanist alternative. *Stud Hist Philos Biol Biomed Sci* 36 (2):421–41.

Bechtel, W. and A. Abrahamsen. 2010. Dynamic mechanistic explanation: Computational modeling of circadian rhythms as an exemplar for cognitive science. *Stud Hist Philos Sci* 41 (3):321–33.

Bechtel, W. and R. C. Richardson. 1993. *Discovering Complexity: Decomposition and Localization as Strategies in Scientific Research.* Princeton, NJ: Princeton University Press.

Beck, S., D. Wojdyla, L. Say, A. P. Betran, M. Merialdi, J. H. Requejo, C. Rubens, R. Menon, and P. F. Van Look. 2010. The worldwide incidence of preterm birth: A systematic review of maternal mortality and morbidity. *Bull World Health Organ* 88 (1):31–8.

Beebee, H., C. Hitchcock, and P. C. Menzies. 2009. *The Oxford Handbook of Causation.* Oxford, UK: Oxford University Press.

Berkman, L. F. and I. Kawachi. 2000. *Social Epidemiology.* New York, NY: Oxford University Press.

Bezold, K. Y., M. K. Karjalainen, M. Hallman, K. Teramo, and L. J. Muglia. 2013. The genomics of preterm birth: From animal models to human studies. *Genome Med* 5 (4):34.

Blackburn, H. and D. Labarthe. 2012. Stories from the evolution of guidelines for causal inference in epidemiologic associations: 1953–1965. *Am J Epidemiol* 176 (12):1071–7.

Blackburn, S. 2016. *The Oxford Dictionary of Philosophy, Oxford Quick Reference (oqr).* New York, NY: Oxford University Press.

Bosch, H. M., A. B. Rosenfield, R. Huston, H. R. Shipman, and F. L. Woodward. 1950. Methemoglobinemia and Minnesota well supplies. *J Am Water Works Assoc* 42 (2):161–70.

Braun, J. M., T. Froehlich, A. Kalkbrenner, C. M. Pfeiffer, Z. Fazili, K. Yolton, and B. P. Lanphear. 2014. Brief report: Are autistic-behaviors in children related to prenatal vitamin use and maternal whole blood folate concentrations? *J Autism Dev Disord* 44 (10):2602–7.

Braunstein, A. and A. Ingrosso. 2016. Inference of causality in epidemics on temporal contact networks. *Sci Rep* 6:27538.

Braveman, P. and L. Gottlieb. 2014. The social determinants of health: It's time to consider the causes of the causes. *Public Health Rep* 129 (Suppl 2):19–31.

Broadbent, A. 2008. The difference between cause and condition. *Proc Aristotelian Soc* 108 (1pt3):355–64.

Broadbent, A. 2011. Inferring causation in epidemiology: Mechanisms, black boxes, and contrasts. In *Causality in the Sciences*, edited by P. M. Illari, F. Russo and J. Williamson, 45–69. Oxford University Press.

Broadbent, A. 2013. *Philosophy of Epidemiology, New Directions in the Philosophy of Science.* Houndmills, UK: Palgrave Macmillan.

Broadbent, A., J. P. Vandenbroucke, and N. Pearce. 2016. Response: Formalism or pluralism? A reply to commentaries on "Causality and causal inference in epidemiology." *Int J Epidemiol* 45 (6):1841–51.

Buck, C. 1975. Popper's philosophy for epidemiologists. *Int J Epidemiol* 4 (3):159–68.

Buck, C. 1989. Problems with the Popperian approach: A response to Pearce and Crawford-Brown. *J Clin Epidemiol* 42 (3):185–7.

Bunge, M. 1979. *Causality and Modern Science*. Dover edition. Cambridge, MA: Harvard University Press.

Carter, K. C. 2003. *The Rise of Causal Concepts of Disease: Case Histories*. Farnham, UK: Ashgate Publishing.

Cartwright, N. 1989. *Nature's Capacities and Their Measurement*. Oxford, UK/New York, NY: Clarendon Press/Oxford University Press.

Cartwright, N. 2004. Causation: One word, many things. *Philos Sci* 71:805–19.

Cartwright, N. 2007. *Hunting Causes and Using Them: Approaches in Philosophy and Economics*. Cambridge, England: Cambridge University Press.

Cartwright, N. 2010. What are randomised controlled trials good for? *Philos Stud* 147 (1):59–70.

Centers for Disease Control and Prevention. 1999. Ten great public health achievements—United States, 1900–1999. *MMWR Morb Mortal Wkly Rep* 48 (12):241–3.

Centers for Disease Control and Prevention. 2011. Ten great public health achievements—United States, 2001–2010. *MMWR Morb Mortal Wkly Rep* 60 (19):619–23.

Chao, H.-K. 2013. *Mechanism and Causality in Biology and Economics*. New York, NY: Springer.

Charlton, B. G. 1996. Attribution of causation in epidemiology: Chain or mosaic?. *J Clin Epidemiol* 49 (1):105–7.

Chez, M. G., T. Dowling, P. B. Patel, P. Khanna, and M. Kominsky. 2007. Elevation of tumor necrosis factor-α in cerebrospinal fluid of autistic children. *Pediatr Neurol* 36 (6):361–5.

Clarke, B., D. Gillies, P. Illari, F. Russo, and J. Williamson. 2013a. The evidence that evidence-based medicine omits. *Prev Med* 57 (6):745–7.

Clarke, B., D. Gillies, P. Illari, F. Russo, and J. Williamson. 2013b. Mechanisms and the evidence hierarchy. *Topoi* 33:339–60.

Claveau, F. 2012. The Russo-Williamson Theses in the social sciences: Causal inference drawing on two types of evidence. *Stud Hist Philos Biol Biomed Sci* 43 (4):806–13.

Cobb, S. 1976. Presidential Address–1976. Social support as a moderator of life stress. *Psychosom Med* 38 (5):300–14.

Collingwood, R. G. 1972. *An Essay on Metaphysics*. Chicago, IL: H. Regnery.

Cooper, W. A., D. C. Lam, S. A. O'Toole, and J. D. Minna. 2013. Molecular biology of lung cancer. *J Thorac Dis* 5 (Suppl 5):S479–90.

Coughlin, S. S. 2014. Toward a road map for global -omics: A primer on -omic technologies. *Am J Epidemiol* 180 (12):1188–95.

Craver, C. F. 2007. *Explaining the Brain*. Oxford, UK: Oxford University Press.

Craver, C. F. and L. Darden. 2013. *In Search of Mechanisms: Discoveries Across the Life Sciences*. Chicago, IL: University of Chicago Press.

Csoka, A. B. 2016. Innovation in medicine: Ignaz the reviled and Egas the regaled. *Med Health Care Philos* 19 (2):163–8.

Damarla, S. R., T. A. Keller, R. K. Kana, V. L. Cherkassky, D. L. Williams, N. J. Minshew, and M. A. Just. 2010. Cortical underconnectivity coupled with preserved visuospatial cognition in autism: Evidence from an fMRI study of an embedded figures task. *Autism Res* 3 (5):273–9.

Dammann, C. E., H. C. Nielsen, and K. L. Carraway 3rd. 2003. Role of neuregulin-1β in the developing lung. *Am J Respir Crit Care Med* 167 (12):1711–6.

Dammann, O. 2015. Epidemiological explanations: A review of A. Broadbent, *Philosophy of Epidemiology*. *Philos Sci* 82 (3):509–19.

Dammann, O. 2016. Causality, mosaics, and the health sciences. *Theor Med Bioeth* 37 (2):161–8.

Dammann, O. 2017. The etiological stance: Explaining illness occurrence. *Perspect Biol Med* 60 (2):151–65.

Dammann, O. 2018. Hill's heuristics and explanatory coherentism in epidemiology. *Am J Epidemiol* 187 (1):1–6.

Dammann, O., S. K. Durum, and A. Leviton. 1999. Modification of the infection-associated risks of preterm birth and white matter damage in the preterm newborn by polymorphisms in the tumor necrosis factor-locus? *Pathogenesis* 1 (3):171–7.

Dammann, O., P. H. Gray, P. Gressens, O. Wolkenhauer, and A Leviton. 2014. Systems epidemiology: What's in a name? *Online J Public Health Inf* 6 (3).

Dammann, O., K. C. Kuban, and A. Leviton. 2002. Perinatal infection, fetal inflammatory response, white matter damage, and cognitive limitations in children born preterm. *Ment Retard Dev Disabil Res Rev* 8 (1):46–50.

Dammann, O. and A. Leviton. 1997. Maternal intrauterine infection, cytokines, and brain damage in the preterm newborn. *Pediatr Res* 42 (1):1–8.

Dammann, O. and A. Leviton. 2004. Inflammatory brain damage in preterm newborns – Dry numbers, wet lab, and causal inference. *Early Hum Dev* 79 (1):1–15.

Dammann, O. and A. Leviton. 2007. Perinatal brain damage causation. *Dev Neurosci* 29 (4–5):280–8.

Dammann, O. and A. Leviton. 2014. Intermittent or sustained systemic inflammation and the preterm brain. *Pediatr Res* 75 (3):376–80.

Dammann, O. and T. M. O'Shea. 2008. Cytokines and perinatal brain damage. *Clin Perinatol* 35 (4):643–63.

Dammann, O., T. Poston, and P. Thagard. 2019. How do medical researchers make causal inferences? In *What Is Scientific Knowledge? An Introduction to Contemporary Epistemology of Science*, edited by K. McCain and K. Kampourakis. New York, NY: Routledge.

Dawid, A. P. 2004. Probability, causality and the empirical world: A Bayes-de Finetti-Popper-Borel synthesis. *Stat Sci* 19 (1):44–57.

Dawid, A. P., D. L. Faigman, and S. E. Fienberg. 2014. Fitting science into legal contexts: Assessing effects of causes or causes of effects? *Sociol Methods Res* 43 (3):359–90.

Deemter, K. v. 2010. *Not Exactly: In Praise of Vagueness*. Oxford, UK: Oxford University Press.

Dekkers, W. and M. O. Rikkert. 2006. What is a genetic cause? The example of Alzheimer's disease. *Med Health Care Philos* 9 (3):273–84.

Di Martino, A., C. Kelly, R. Grzadzinski, X. N. Zuo, M. Mennes, M. A. Mairena, C. Lord, F. X. Castellanos, and M. P. Milham. 2011. Aberrant striatal functional connectivity in children with autism. *Biol Psychiatry* 69 (9):847–56.

Doll, R. 2002. Proof of causality: Deduction from epidemiological observation. *Perspect Biol Med* 45 (4):499–515.

Dowe, P. 1995. Causality and conserved quantities – A reply. *Philos Sci* 62 (2): 321–33.

Dowe, P. 2000. *Physical Causation, Cambridge Studies in Probability, Induction, and Decision Theory.* Cambridge, England: Cambridge University Press.

Dowe, P. 2009. Causal process theories. In *The Oxford Handbook of Causation*, edited by H. Beebee, C. Hitchcock and P. Menzies, 213–33. Oxford, UK: Oxford University Press.

Du, X., B. Fleiss, H. Li, B. D'Angelo, Y. Sun, C. Zhu, H. Hagberg, O. Levy, C. Mallard, and X. Wang. 2011. Systemic stimulation of TLR2 impairs neonatal mouse brain development. *PLOS ONE* 6 (5):e19583.

du Plessis, A. J. and J. J. Volpe. 2002. Perinatal brain injury in the preterm and term newborn. *Curr Opin Neurol* 15 (2):151–7.

Dupré, J. 2013. Living causes. *Aristotelian Society Supplementary, LXXXVII*:19–37.

Eells, E. 1991. *c.* Cambridge, England: Cambridge University Press.

Eisenberger, N. I. and S. W. Cole. 2012. Social neuroscience and health: Neurophysiological mechanisms linking social ties with physical health. *Nat Neurosci* 15 (5):669–74.

Eklind, S., C. Mallard, P. Arvidsson, and H. Hagberg. 2005. Lipopolysaccharide induces both a primary and a secondary phase of sensitization in the developing rat brain. *Pediatr Res* 58 (1):112–6.

Emmert-Streib, F. and M. Dehmer. 2010. *Medical Biostatistics for Complex Diseases.* Weinheim, Germany: Wiley-Blackwell.

Engel, G. L. 1977. The need for a new medical model: A challenge for biomedicine. *Science* 196 (4286):129–36.

Engel, G. L. 1980. The clinical application of the biopsychosocial model. *Am J Psychiatry* 137 (5):535–44.

Erdei, C. and O. Dammann. 2014. The perfect storm: Preterm birth, neurodevelopmental mechanisms, and autism causation. *Perspect Biol Med* 57 (4):470–81.

Evans, A. S. 1978. Causation and disease: A chronological journey. *Am J Epidemiol* 108 (4):249–58.

Evans, A. S. 1993. *Causation and Disease: A Chronological Journey.* New York, NY: Plenum Publishing.

Fagot-Largeault, A. 1989. *Les causes de la mort: Histoire naturelle et facteurs de risque.* Paris, France: Institut interdisciplinaire d'études épistémologiques.

Fava, G. A. and N. Sonino. 2008. The biopsychosocial model thirty years later. *Psychother Psychosom* 77 (1):1–2.

Favrais, G., Y. van de Looij, B. Fleiss, N. Ramanantsoa, P. Bonnin, G. Stoltenburg-Didinger, A. Lacaud et al. 2011. Systemic inflammation disrupts the developmental program of white matter. *Ann Neurol* 70 (4):550–65.

Faye, J. 2018. Backward causation. In *The Stanford Encyclopedia of Philosophy (Summer 2018 ed.)*, edited by E. N. Zalta.

Fetzer, J. 2017. Carl Hempel. In *The Stanford Encyclopedia of Philosophy* edited by E. N. Zalta.

Fiorentino, A. R. and O. Dammann. 2015. Evidence, disease, and causation: An epidemiologic perspective on the Russo-Williamson thesis. *Studies Hist Philos Biol Biomed Sci* 54:1–9.

Flanagan, R. and O. Dammann. 2018. The epistemological weight of randomized-controlled trials depends on their results. *Perspect Biol Med* 61 (2):157–73.

Flanders, W. D., M. Klein, L. A. Darrow, M. J. Strickland, S. E. Sarnat, J. A. Sarnat, L. A. Waller, A. Winquist, and P. E. Tolbert. 2011a. A method for detection of residual confounding in time-series and other observational studies. *Epidemiology* 22 (1):59–67.

Flanders, W. D., M. Klein, L. A. Darrow, M. J. Strickland, S. E. Sarnat, J. A. Sarnat, L. A. Waller, A. Winquist, and P. E. Tolbert. 2011b. A method to detect residual confounding in spatial and other observational studies. *Epidemiology* 22 (6):823–6.

Fleck, L. 1935 (2012). *Entstehung und Entwicklung einer wissenschaftlichen Tatsache, wissenschaft 312*. Frankfurt, Germany: Suhrkamp.

Flier, F. J. and P. F. de Vries Robbé. 1999. Nosology and causal necessity; the relation between defining a disease and discovering its necessary cause. *Theor Med Bioeth* 20 (6):577–88.

Frank, C., M. Faber, and K. Stark. 2016. Causal or not: Applying the Bradford Hill aspects of evidence to the association between Zika virus and microcephaly. *EMBO Mol Med* 8 (4):305–7.

Friedman, M. 1974. Explanation and scientific understanding. *J Philos* 71 (1):5–19.

Galea, S., M. Riddle, and G. A. Kaplan. 2010. Causal thinking and complex system approaches in epidemiology. *Int J Epidemiol* 39 (1):97–106.

Garson, J. 2013. The functional sense of mechanism. *Philos Sci* 80 (3):317–33.

Gasking, D. 1955. Causation and recipes. *Minds Mach J Artif Intell, Philos Cogn Sci* 64 (256):479–87.

Gaugler, T., L. Klei, S. J. Sanders, C. A. Bodea, A. P. Goldberg, A. B. Lee, M. Mahajan et al. 2014. Most genetic risk for autism resides with common variation. *Nat Genet* 46 (8):881–5.

Gelman, A. 2011. Causality and statistical learning. *Am J Sociol* 117 (3):955–66.

Gidaya, N. B., B. K. Lee, I. Burstyn, M. Yudell, E. L. Mortensen, and C. J. Newschaffer. 2014. *In utero* exposure to selective serotonin reuptake inhibitors and risk for autism spectrum disorder. *J Autism Dev Disord* 44 (10):2558–67.

Giere, R. N. 1997. *Understanding Scientific Reasoning*. 4th ed. Fort Worth, TX: Harcourt, Brace, Jovanovich.

Gifford, F. 2011. *Philosophy of Medicine. 1st ed., Handbook of the Philosophy of Science*. Boston, MA: Elsevier/North Holland.

Gilles, F., P. Gressens, O. Dammann, and A. Leviton. 2018. Hypoxia-ischemia is not an antecedent of most preterm brain damage: The illusion of validity. *Dev Med Child Neurol* 60 (2):120–25.

Gillies, D. 2011. The Russo-Williamson thesis and the question of whether smoking causes heart disease. In *Causality in the Sciences*, edited by P. M. Illari, F. Russo and J. Williamson, 110–25. Oxford, UK: Oxford University Press.

Glass, T. A., S. N. Goodman, M. A. Hernan, and J. M. Samet. 2013. Causal inference in public health. *Annu Rev Public Health* 34:61–75.

Gleeson, M., N. C. Bishop, D. J. Stensel, M. R. Lindley, S. S. Mastana, and M. A. Nimmo. 2011. The anti-inflammatory effects of exercise: Mechanisms and implications for the prevention and treatment of disease. *Nat Rev Immunol* 11 (9):607–15.

Glennan, S. S. 1996. Mechanisms and the nature of causation. *Erkenntnis* 44:49–71.

Glennan, S. 2002. Rethinking mechanistic explanation. *Philos Sci* 69 (S3):S342–53.

Glennan, S. 2008. Mechanisms. In *The Routledge Companion to Philosophy of Science*, edited by S. Psillos and M. Curd, 376–84. London: Routledge.

Glennan, S. 2011. Singular and general causal relations: A mechanism perspective. In *Causality in the Sciences*, edited by P. Illari, F. Russo and J. Williamson, 789–844. Oxford, UK: Oxford University Press.

Godfrey-Smith, P. 2009. Causal pluralism. In *The Oxford Handbook of Causation*, edited by H. Beebee, C. Hitchcock and P. Menzies, 326–37. Oxford, UK: Oxford University Press.

Gopnik, A. and L. Schulz. 2007. *Causal Learning: Psychology, Philosophy, and Computation*. Oxford, UK: Oxford University Press.

Gordis, L. 2014. *Epidemiology*. 5th ed. Philadelphia, PA: Elsevier Saunders.

Gorrindo, P., K. C. Williams, E. B. Lee, L. S. Walker, S. G. McGrew, and P. Levitt. 2012. Gastrointestinal dysfunction in autism: Parental report, clinical evaluation, and associated factors. *Autism Res* 5 (2):101–8.

Goyal, D. K. and J. A. Miyan. 2014. Neuro-immune abnormalities in autism and their relationship with the environment: A variable insult model for autism. *Front Endocrinol (Lausanne)* 5:29.

Greenland, S. 1988. Probability versus Popper: An elaboration of the insufficiency of current Popperian approaches for epidemiologic analysis. In *Causal Inference*, edited by K. J. Rothman. Chestnut Hill, MA: Epidemiology Resources, Inc.

Greenland, S. 1998. Induction versus Popper: Substance versus semantics. *Int J Epidemiol* 27 (4):543–8.

Greenland, S. 1999. Relation of probability of causation to relative risk and doubling dose: A methodologic error that has become a social problem. *Am J Public Health* 89 (8):1166–9.

Greenland, S. and B. Brumback. 2002. An overview of relations among causal modelling methods. *Int J Epidemiol* 31 (5):1030–7.

Haack, S. 2004. An epistemologist among the epidemiologists. *Epidemiology* 15 (5):521–2; author reply 527–8.

Haack, S. 1993. *Evidence and Inquiry: Towards Reconstruction in Epistemology*. Oxford, UK: Blackwell.

Hack, M., H. G. Taylor, M. Schluchter, L. Andreias, D. Drotar, and N. Klein. 2009. Behavioral outcomes of extremely low birth weight children at age 8 years. *J Dev Behav Pediatr* 30 (2):122–30.

Hagberg, H., O. Dammann, C. Mallard, and A. Leviton. 2004. Preconditioning and the developing brain. *Semin Perinatol* 28:389–95.

Hagberg, H., P. Gressens, and C. Mallard. 2012. Inflammation during fetal and neonatal life: Implications for neurologic and neuropsychiatric disease in children and adults. *Ann Neurol* 71 (4):444–57.

Hallmayer, J., S. Cleveland, A. Torres, J. Phillips, B. Cohen, T. Torigoe, J. Miller et al. 2011. Genetic heritability and shared environmental factors among twin pairs with autism. *Arch Gen Psychiatry* 68 (11):1095–102.

Happé, F., A. Ronald, and R. Plomin. 2006. Time to give up on a single explanation for autism. *Nat Neurosci* 9 (10):1218–20.

Harman, G. H. 1965. The inference to the best explanation. *Philos Rev* 74 (1):88–95.

Healey, R. 2009. Causation in quantum mechanics. In *The Oxford Handbook of Causation*, edited by H. Beebee, C. Hitchcock and P. Menzies, 673–86. Oxford, UK: Oxford University Press.

Hecht, S. S. 2012. Lung carcinogenesis by tobacco smoke. *Int J Cancer* 131 (12): 2724–32.

Hempel, C. G. and P. Oppenheim. 1948. Studies in the logic of explanation. *Philos Sci* 15 (2):135–75.

Hernán, M. A. 2004. A definition of causal effect for epidemiological research. *J Epidemiol Community Health* 58 (4):265–71.

Hernán, M. A., S. Hernández-Diaz, M. M. Werler, and A. A. Mitchell. 2002. Causal knowledge as a prerequisite for confounding evaluation: An application to birth defects epidemiology. *Am J Epidemiol* 155 (2):176–84.

Hernán, M. A. and J. M. Robins. 2006a. Estimating causal effects from epidemiologic data. *J Epidemiol Community Health* 60:578–86.

Hernán, M. A. and J. M. Robins. 2006b. Instruments for causal inference: An epidemiologist's dream? *Epidemiology* 17 (4):360–72.

Hernán, M. A. and J. M. Robins. 2020. *Causal Inference: What If*. Boca Raton, FL: Chapman & Hall/CRC.

Hill, A. B. 1953. Observation and experiment. *N Engl J Med* 248 (24):995–1001.

Hill, A. B. 1965. The environment and disease: Association or causation? *Proc R Soc Med* 58:295–300.

Hofer, T., H. Przyrembel, and S. Verleger. 2004. New evidence for the theory of the stork. *Paediatr Perinat Epidemiol* 18 (1):88–92.

Höfler, M. 2005. The Bradford Hill considerations on causality: A counterfactual perspective. *Emerg Themes Epidemiol* 2:11.

Höfler, M. 2006. Getting causal considerations back on the right track. *Emerg Themes Epidemiol* 3:8.

Howson, C. and P. Urbach. 1993. *Scientific Reasoning: The Bayesian Approach*. 2nd ed. Chicago, IL: Open Court.

Huguet, G., E. Ey, and T. Bourgeron. 2013. The genetic landscapes of autism spectrum disorders. *Annu Rev Genomics Hum Genet* 14:191–213.

Hulley, S., D. Grady, T. Bush, C. Furberg, D. Herrington, B. Riggs, and E. Vittinghoff. 1998. Randomized trial of estrogen plus progestin for secondary prevention of coronary heart disease in postmenopausal women. Heart and Estrogen/progestin Replacement Study (HERS) Research Group. *JAMA* 280 (7):605–13.

Illari, P. M. 2011. Mechanistic evidence: Disambiguating the Russo–Williamson thesis. *Int Stud Philos Sci* 25:139–57.

Illari, P. M. and J. Williamson. 2012. What is a mechanism? Thinking about mechanisms *across* the sciences. *Eur J Phil Sci* 2:119–35.

Illari, P. M. and F. Russo. 2014. *Causality: Philosophical Theory Meets Scientific Practice*. Oxford, UK: Oxford University Press.

Illari, P. M., F. Russo, and J. Williamson. 2011. *Causality in the Sciences*. Oxford, UK: Oxford University Press.

Imbens, G. and D. B. Rubin. 2015. *Causal Inference for Statistics, Social, and Biomedical Sciences – An Introduction*. New York, NY: Cambridge University Press.

Ioannidis, J. P. 2015. Exposure-wide epidemiology: Revisiting Bradford Hill. *Stat Med* 35 (11):1749–62.

Iossifov, I., B. J. O'Roak, S. J. Sanders, M. Ronemus, N. Krumm, D. Levy, H. A. Stessman et al. 2014. The contribution of *de novo* coding mutations to autism spectrum disorder. *Nature* 515 (7526):216–21.

Jacobsen, M. 1976. Against Popperized epidemiology. *Int J Epidemiol* 5 (1):9–11.

Jaffer, U., R. G. Wade, and T. Gourlay. 2010. Cytokines in the systemic inflammatory response syndrome: A review. *HSR Proc Intensive Care Cardiovasc Anesth* 2 (3):161–75.

Jenkins, D., C. McCuaig, B. A. Drolet, D. Siegel, S. Adams, J. A. Lawson, and O. Wargon. 2016. Tuberous sclerosis complex associated with vascular anomalies or overgrowth. *Pediatr Dermatol* 33 (5):536–42.

Joffe, M. 2013. The concept of causation in biology. *Erkenntnis: An Int J Anal Philos* 78 (2):179–97.

Johnson, S., C. Hollis, P. Kochhar, E. Hennessy, D. Wolke, and N. Marlow. 2010. Autism spectrum disorders in extremely preterm children. *J Pediatr* 156 (4):525–31 e2.

Just, M. A., T. A. Keller, V. L. Malave, R. K. Kana, and S. Varma. 2012. Autism as a neural systems disorder: A theory of frontal-posterior underconnectivity. *Neurosci Biobehav Rev* 36 (4):1292–313.

Kapitanovic Vidak, H., T. Catela Ivkovic, M. Jokic, R. Spaventi, and S. Kapitanovic. 2012. The association between proinflammatory cytokine polymorphisms and cerebral palsy in very preterm infants. *Cytokine* 58 (1):57–64.

Karhausen, L. R. 1995. The poverty of Popperian epidemiology. *Int J Epidemiol* 24 (5):869–74.

Karmiloff-Smith, A. 1998. Development itself is the key to understanding developmental disorders. *Trends Cog Sci* 2 (10):389–98.

Keil, K. P. and P. J. Lein. 2016. DNA methylation: A mechanism linking environmental chemical exposures to risk of autism spectrum disorders? *Environ Epigenet* 2 (1).

Kelleher, J. D., B. M. Namee, and A. D'Arcy. 2015. *Fundamentals of Machine Learning for Predictive Data Analytics: Algorithms, Worked Examples, and Case Studies*. Cambridge, MA: MIT Press.

Kelly, M. P., R. S. Kelly, and F. Russo. 2014. The integration of social, behavioral, and biological mechanisms in models of pathogenesis. *Perspect Biol Med* 57 (3):308–28.

Kerry, R., T. E. Eriksen, S. A. Lie, S. D. Mumford, and R. L. Anjum. 2012. Causation and evidence-based practice: An ontological review. *J Eval Clin Pract* 18 (5):1006–12.

Kerschensteiner, M., E. Meinl, and R. Hohlfeld. 2009. Neuro-immune crosstalk in CNS diseases. *Neuroscience* 158 (3):1122–32.

Khoury, M. J., T. H. Beaty, and B. H. Cohen. 1993. *Fundamentals of Genetic Epidemiology*. New York, Oxford: Oxford University Press, p.12.

Kincaid, H. 2011. Causal modelling, mechanism, and probability in epidemiology. In *Causality in the Sciences*, edited by P. Illari, F. Russo and J. Williamson, 70–90. Oxford, UK: Oxford University Press.

Kitcher, P. 1981. Explanatory unification. *Philos Sci* 48 (4):507–31.

Kitcher, P. 1989. Explanatory unification and the causal structure of the world. In *Scientific Explanation*, edited by P. Kitcher and W. Salmon, 410–505. Minneapolis, MN: University of Minnesota Press.

Kleinberg, S. and G. Hripcsak. 2011. A review of causal inference for biomedical informatics. *J Biomed Inform* 44 (6):1102–12.

Krieger, N. 1994. Epidemiology and the web of causation: Has anyone seen the spider? *Soc Sci Med* 39 (7):887–903.

Krieger, N. 2011. *Epidemiology and the People's Health: Theory and Context*. New York, NY: Oxford University Press.

Kuban, K. C., T. M. O'Shea, E. N. Allred, H. Tager-Flusberg, D. J. Goldstein, and A. Leviton. 2009. Positive screening on the Modified Checklist for Autism in Toddlers (M-CHAT) in extremely low gestational age newborns. *J Pediatr* 154 (4):535–40 e1.

Kundi, M. 2006. Causality and the interpretation of epidemiologic evidence. *Environ Health Perspect* 114 (7):969–74.

La Caze, A. 2013. Why randomized interventional studies. *J Med Philos* 38 (4):352–68.

Lai, M. C., M. V. Lombardo, and S. Baron-Cohen. 2014. Autism. *Lancet* 383 (9920):896–910.

Lampi, K. M., L. Lehtonen, P. L. Tran, A. Suominen, V. Lehti, P. N. Banerjee, M. Gissler, A. S. Brown, and A. Sourander. 2012. Risk of autism spectrum disorders in low birth weight and small for gestational age infants. *J Pediatr* 161 (5):830–6.

Lawson, A. B. 2012. Bayesian point event modeling in spatial and environmental epidemiology. *Stat Methods Med Res* 21 (5):509–29.

Lerner, B. H. 2005. Last-ditch medical therapy – Revisiting lobotomy. *N Engl J Med* 353 (2):119–21.

Leviton, A. and P. Gressens. 2007. Neuronal damage accompanies perinatal white-matter damage. *Trends Neurosci* 30 (9):473–8.

Lewis, D. 1973. Causation. *J Philos* 70:556–67.

Lewis, D., ed. 1986. Causal explanation. In *Philosophical Papers*, Vol. 214–40. Oxford, UK: Oxford University Press.

Li, J., O. Baud, T. Vartanian, J. J. Volpe, and P. A. Rosenberg. 2005. Peroxynitrite generated by inducible nitric oxide synthase and NADPH oxidase mediates microglial toxicity to oligodendrocytes. *Proc Natl Acad Sci USA* 102 (28):9936–41.

Lilienfeld, A. M. 1957. Epidemiological methods and inferences in studies of non-infectious diseases. *Public Health Rep* 72 (1):51–60.

Lilienfeld, A. M. 1959. On the methodology of investigations of etiologic factors in chronic diseases: Some comments. *J Chronic Dis* 10 (1):41–6.

Limperopoulos, C., H. Bassan, N. R. Sullivan, J. S. Soul, R. L. Robertson, Jr., M. Moore, S. A. Ringer, J. J. Volpe, and A. J. du Plessis. 2008. Positive screening for autism in ex-preterm infants: Prevalence and risk factors. *Pediatrics* 121 (4):758–65.

Lin, C. Y., Y. C. Chang, S. T. Wang, T. Y. Lee, C. F. Lin, and C. C. Huang. 2010. Altered inflammatory responses in preterm children with cerebral palsy. *Ann Neurol* 68 (2):204–12.

Lipton, P. 1991. *Inference to the Best Explanation, Philosophical Issues in Science Series*. London, UK: Routledge.

Lipton, P. 1992. Causation outside the law. In *Jurisprudence: Cambridge Essays*, edited by H. Gross and R. Harrison, 127–48. Oxford, UK: Oxford University Press.

Lipton, P. 2004. *Inference to the Best Explanation*. 2nd ed. London, UK: Routledge/ Taylor & Francis Group.

Lipton, R. and T. Ødegaard. 2005. Causal thinking and causal language in epidemiology: It's in the details. *Epidemiol Perspect Innov* 2:8.

Little, R. J. and D. B. Rubin. 2000. Causal effects in clinical and epidemiological studies via potential outcomes: Concepts and analytical approaches. *Annu Rev Public Health* 21:121–45.

Lucas, R. M. and A. J. McMichael. 2005. Association or causation: Evaluating links between "environment and disease." *Bull World Health Organ* 83 (10):792–5.

Luthra, S. 2015. The scientific foundation, rationale and argument for a nonfrequentist Bayesian analysis in clinical trials in coronary artery disease. *Heart Lung Circ* 24 (6):614–6.

Lyall, K., R. J. Schmidt, and I. Hertz-Picciotto. 2014. Maternal lifestyle and environmental risk factors for autism spectrum disorders. *Int J Epidemiol* 43 (2):443–64.

Machamer, P. K., L. Darden, and C. F. Craver. 2000. Thinking about mechanisms. *Philos Sci* 67:1–25.

Mackie, J. L. 1965. Causes and conditions. *Am Philos Q* 2 (4):245–64.

Mackie, J. L. 1974. *The Cement of the Universe; A Study of Causation, The Clarendon Library of Logic and Philosophy*. Oxford, UK: Clarendon Press.

Maclure, M. 1985. Popperian refutation in epidemiology. *Am J Epidemiol* 121 (3):343–50.

MacMahon, B. and T. F. Pugh. 1970. *Epidemiology; Principles and Methods*. Boston, MA: Little, Brown and Company.

Mahoney, A. D., B. Minter, K. Burch, and J. Stapel-Wax. 2013. Autism spectrum disorders and prematurity: A review across gestational age subgroups. *Adv Neonatal Care* 13 (4):247–51.

Main, C., B. Knight, T. Moxham, R. Gabriel Sanchez, L. M. Sanchez Gomez, M. Roque i Figuls, and X. Bonfill Cosp. 2013. Hormone therapy for preventing cardiovascular disease in post-menopausal women. *Cochrane Database Syst Rev* 4:CD002229.

Malaeb, S. and O. Dammann. 2009. Fetal inflammatory response and brain injury in the preterm newborn. *J Child Neurol* 24 (9):1119–26.

Maldonado, G. and S. Greenland. 2002. Estimating causal effects. *Int J Epidemiol* 31 (2):422–9.

Mallard, C. and H. Hagberg. 2007. Inflammation-induced preconditioning in the immature brain. *Semin Fetal Neonatal Med* 12 (4):280–6.

Marshall, B. D. and S. Galea. 2015. Formalizing the role of agent-based modeling in causal inference and epidemiology. *Am J Epidemiol* 181 (2):92–9.

Martin, J. A., B. E. Hamilton, and M. J. Osterman. 2014. Births in the United States, 2013. *NCHS Data Brief* (175):1–8.

Mayr, E. 1961. Cause and effect in biology. *Science* 134:1501–6.

McDowell, I. 2008. From risk factors to explanation in public health. *J Public Health (Oxf)* 30 (3):219–23.

Mercuri, M. and B. S. Baigrie. 2016. Interpreting risk as evidence of causality: Lessons learned from a legal case to determine medical malpractice. *J Eval Clin Pract* 22 (4):515–21.

Meyer, U., J. Feldon, and O. Dammann. 2011. Schizophrenia and autism: Both shared and disorder-specific pathogenesis via perinatal inflammation? *Pediatr Res* 69 (5 Pt 2):26R–33R.

Miettinen, O. S. 1985. *Theoretical Epidemiology*. New York, NY: John Wiley & Sons.

Miettinen, O. S. and K. M. Flegel. 2003. Elementary concepts of medicine: VI. Genesis of illness: Pathogenesis, aetiogenesis. *J Eval Clin Pract* 9 (3):325–7.

Miettinen, O. S. and I. Karp. 2012. *Epidemiological research: An introduction*. Dordrecht, Netherlands: Springer.

Mill, J. S. 1856. *A System of Logic*. 4th ed. London, UK: John W. Parker & Son.

Minshew, N. J. and T. A. Keller. 2010. The nature of brain dysfunction in autism: Functional brain imaging studies. *Curr Opin Neurol* 23 (2):124–30.

Monaghan, K. G., G. L. Feldman, G. E. Palomaki, E. B. Spector, Ashkenazi Jewish Reproductive Screening Working Group, and Molecular Subcommittee of the ACMG Laboratory Quality Assurance Committee. 2008. Technical standards and guidelines for reproductive screening in the Ashkenazi Jewish population. *Genet Med* 10 (1):57–72.

Morabia, A. 1991. On the origin of Hill's causal criteria. *Epidemiology* 2 (5): 367–9.

Morabia, A. 2013. Hume, Mill, Hill, and the sui generis epidemiologic approach to causal inference. *Am J Epidemiol* 178 (10):1526–32.

Morabia, A. 2014. *Enigmas of Health and Disease: How Epidemiology Helps Unravel Scientific Mysteries*. New York, NY: Columbia University Press.

Morgan, J. T., G. Chana, C. A. Pardo, C. Achim, K. Semendeferi, J. Buckwalter, E. Courchesne, and I. P. Everall. 2010. Microglial activation and increased microglial density observed in the dorsolateral prefrontal cortex in autism. *Biol Psychiatry* 68 (4):368–76.

Mumford, S. 2009. Causal powers and capacities. In *The Oxford Handbook of Causation*, edited by H. Beebee, C. Hitchcock and P. Menzies, 265–78. Oxford, UK: Oxford University Press.

Mumford, S. and R. L. Anjum, eds. 2011a. *Getting Causes from Powers*. Oxford, UK: Oxford University Press.

Mumford, S. and R. L. Anjum. 2011b. Passing powers around. In *Getting Causes from Powers*, 1–18. Oxford, UK: Oxford University Press.

Negrini, S., F. Pappalardo, G. Murdaca, F. Indiveri, and F. Puppo. 2016. The antiphospholipid syndrome: From pathophysiology to treatment. *Clin Exp Med* 17 (3):257–67.

Nicholson, D. J. 2012. The concept of mechanism in biology. *Stud Hist Philos Biol Biomed Sci* 43 (1):152–63.

Nordenfelt, L. and B. I. B. Lindahl. 1984. *Health, Disease, and Causal Explanations in Medicine, Philosophy and Medicine.* Dordrecht, Netherlands: Kluwer Academic.

Norell, S. 1984. Models of causation in epidemiology. In *Health, Disease, and Causal Explanations in Medicine,* edited by L. Nordenfelt and B. I. B. Lindahl, 129–35. Dordrecht, Netherlands: D. Reidel Publishing.

Novack, D. H., O. Cameron, E. Epel, R. Ader, S. R. Waldstein, S. Levenstein, M. H. Antoni, and A. R. Wainer. 2007. Psychosomatic medicine: The scientific foundation of the biopsychosocial model. *Acad Psychiatry* 31 (5):388–401.

OCEBM Levels of Evidence Working Group. 2011. The Oxford 2011 Levels of Evidence. Oxford, UK: Oxford Centre for Evidence-Based Medicine.

Old, L. J. 1985. Tumor necrosis factor (TNF). *Science* 230 (4726):630–2.

Oleckno, W. A. 2008. *Epidemiology: Concepts and Methods.* Long Grove, IL: Waveland Press.

Olsson, E. J. 2005. *Against Coherence: Truth, Probability, and Justification.* Oxford, UK: Oxford University Press.

Ostergren, P. O., B. S. Hanson, I. Balogh, J. Ektor-Andersen, A. Isacsson, P. Orbaek, J. Winkel, S. O. Isacsson, and Group Malmo Shoulder Neck Study. 2005. Incidence of shoulder and neck pain in a working population: Effect modification between mechanical and psychosocial exposures at work? Results from a one year follow up of the Malmo shoulder and neck study cohort. *J Epidemiol Community Health* 59 (9):721–8.

Ostrer, H. 2001. A genetic profile of contemporary Jewish populations. *Nat Rev Genet* 2 (11):891–8.

Papineau, D. 1994. The virtues of randomization. *Br J Philos Sci* 45 (2):437–50.

Parascandola, M. and D. L. Weed. 2001. Causation in epidemiology. *J Epidemiol Community Health* 55 (12):905–12.

Pascal, A., P. Govaert, A. Oostra, G. Naulaers, E. Ortibus, and C. Van den Broeck. 2018. Neurodevelopmental outcome in very preterm and very-low-birthweight infants born over the past decade: A meta-analytic review. *Dev Med Child Neurol* 60 (4):342–55.

Patterson, P. H. 2009. Immune involvement in schizophrenia and autism: Etiology, pathology and animal models. *Behav Brain Res* 204 (2):313–21.

Pearce, N. 1990. White swans, black ravens, and lame ducks: Necessary and sufficient causes in epidemiology. *Epidemiology* 1 (1):47–50.

Pearce, N. 2012. Lost in translation. *Int J Epidemiol* 41 (3):893–5.

Pearce, N. and D. Crawford-Brown. 1989. Critical discussion in epidemiology: Problems with the Popperian approach. *J Clin Epidemiol* 42 (3):177–84.

Pearce, N. and F. Merletti. 2006. Complexity, simplicity, and epidemiology. *Int J Epidemiol* 35 (3):515–9.

Pearl, J. 1988. Embracing causality in default reasoning. *Artif Intell* 35 (2):259–71.

Pearl, J. 2000. *Causality: Models, Reasoning, and Inference.* Cambridge, England: Cambridge University Press.

Pearson, K. 1900. *The Grammar of Science.* 2nd ed. London, UK: A and C Black.

Peirce, C. S. S. 1906. Prolegomena to an apology for pragmaticism. *The Monist* 16:492–546.

Penn, N., E. Oteng-Ntim, L. L. Oakley, and P. Doyle. 2014. Ethnic variation in stillbirth risk and the role of maternal obesity: Analysis of routine data from a London maternity unit. *BMC Pregnancy Childbirth* 14 (1):404.

Petersen, M. L., S. E. Sinisi, and M. J. van der Laan. 2006. Estimation of direct causal effects. *Epidemiology* 17 (3):276–84.

Pfeifer, G. P. and A. Besaratinia. 2012. UV wavelength-dependent DNA damage and human non-melanoma and melanoma skin cancer. *Photochem Photobiol Sci* 11 (1):90–7.

Philippe, P. and O. Mansi. 1998. Nonlinearity in the epidemiology of complex health and disease processes. *Theor Med Bioeth* 19 (6):591–607.

Phillips, C. V. and K. J. Goodman. 2004. The missed lessons of Sir Austin Bradford Hill. *Epidemiol Perspect Innov* 1 (1):3.

Phillips, C. V. and K. J. Goodman. 2006. Causal criteria and counterfactuals; nothing more (or less) than scientific common sense. *Emerg Themes Epidemiol* 3:5.

Poole, C. 2001. Causal values. *Epidemiology* 12 (2):139–41.

Poston, T. 2014. *Reason and Explanation: A Defense of Explanatory Coherentism, Palgrave Innovations in Philosophy.* Basingstoke, UK: Palgrave Macmillan.

Räisänen, U., M. J. Bekkers, P. Boddington, S. Sarangi, and A. Clarke. 2006. The causation of disease – The practical and ethical consequences of competing explanations. *Med Health Care Philos* 9 (3):293–306.

Rasmussen, S. A., D. J. Jamieson, M. A. Honein, and L. R. Petersen. 2016. Zika virus and birth defects – Reviewing the evidence for causality. *N Engl J Med* 374 (20):1981–7.

Raymond, L. J., R. C. Deth, and N. V. Ralston. 2014. Potential role of selenoenzymes and antioxidant metabolism in relation to autism etiology and pathology. *Autism Res Treat* 2014:164938.

Reichenbach, H. 1957. *The Philosophy of Space and Time.* New York, NY: Dover.

Reiss, J. 2011. Third time's a charm: Causation, science, and Wittgensteinian pluralism. In *Causality in the Sciences*, edited by P. M. Illari, F. Russo and J. Williamson. Oxford, UK: Oxford University Press.

Renton, A. 1994. Epidemiology and causation: A realist view. *J Epidemiol Community Health* 48 (1):79–85.

Rescher, N. 1996. *Process Metaphysics: An Introduction to Process Philosophy, SUNY Series in Philosophy.* Albany, NY: State University of New York Press.

Rescher, N. 2000. *Process Philosophy: A Survey of Basic Issues.* Pittsburgh, PA: University of Pittsburgh Press.

Richiardi, L., R. Bellocco, and D. Zugna. 2013. Mediation analysis in epidemiology: Methods, interpretation and bias. *Int J Epidemiol* 42 (5):1511–9.

Ridker, P. M., N. R. Cook, I. M. Lee, D. Gordon, J. M. Gaziano, J. E. Manson, C. H. Hennekens, and J. E. Buring. 2005. A randomized trial of low-dose aspirin in the primary prevention of cardiovascular disease in women. *N Engl J Med* 352 (13):1293–304.

Rizzi, D. A. 1994. Causal reasoning and the diagnostic process. *Theor Med* 15 (3):315–33.

Rizzi, D. A. and S. A. Pedersen. 1992. Causality in medicine: Towards a theory and terminology. *Theor Med* 13 (3):233–54.

Robins, J. M. 2001. Data, design, and background knowledge in etiologic inference. *Epidemiology* 12 (3):313–20.

Rodriguez, J. I. and J. K. Kern. 2011. Evidence of microglial activation in autism and its possible role in brain underconnectivity. *Neuron Glia Biol* 7 (2–4):205–13.

Ronemus, M., I. Iossifov, D. Levy, and M. Wigler. 2014. The role of *de novo* mutations in the genetics of autism spectrum disorders. *Nat Rev Genet* 15 (2):133–41.

Rose, G. 1985. Sick individuals and sick populations. *Int J Epidemiol* 14 (1):32–8.

Rose, G. A. 1992. *The Strategy of Preventive Medicine*. Oxford, UK: Oxford University Press.

Ross, J. R. 1965. *Constraints on Variables in Syntax*. Cambridge, MA: Department of Modern Languages and Linguistics, Massachusetts Institute of Technology.

Rossignol, D. A. and R. E. Frye. 2012. A review of research trends in physiological abnormalities in autism spectrum disorders: Immune dysregulation, inflammation, oxidative stress, mitochondrial dysfunction and environmental toxicant exposures. *Mol Psychiatry* 17 (4):389–401.

Rothman, K. J. 1976. Causes. *Am J Epidemiol* 104:87–92.

Rothman, K. J. 1981. Induction and latent periods. *Am J Epidemiol* 114 (2):253–9.

Rothman, K. J. 1986. *Modern Epidemiology*. Boston, MA: Little, Brown & Company.

Rothman, K.J., ed. 1988. *Causal Inference*. Chestnut Hill, MA: Epidemiology Resources, Inc.

Rothman, K. J. and S. Greenland. 1998. *Modern Epidemiology*. 2nd ed. Philadelphia, PA: Lippincott-Raven.

Rothman, K. J. and S. Greenland. 2005. Hill's criteria for causality. In *Encyclopedia of Biostatistics,* Online. Doi: 10.1002/0470011815.b2a03072.

Rothman, K. J., S Greenland, and T. L. Lash. 2008a. Types of epidemiologic studies. In *Modern Epidemiology,* edited by K. J. Rothman, S. Greenland and T. L. Lash, 87–99. Philadelphia, PA: Wolters Kluwer/Lippincott Williams & Wilkins.

Rothman, K. J., S. Greenland, and T. L. Lash. 2008b. *Modern Epidemiology*. 3rd ed. Philadelphia, PA: Wolters Kluwer Health/Lippincott Williams & Wilkins.

Rothman, K. J., S. Greenland, C. Poole, and T. L. Lash. 2008c. Causation and causal inference. In *Modern Epidemiology,* edited by K. J. Rothman, S. Greenland and T. L. Lash, 5–31. Philadelphia, PA: Lippincott Williams & Wilkins.

Rothman, K. J. and B. E. Mahon. 2004. Confounding and effect-measure modification in the evaluation of immunogenic agents. *Eur J Epidemiol* 19 (3):205–7.

Rousset, C. I., S. Chalon, S. Cantagrel, S. Bodard, C. Andres, P. Gressens, and E. Saliba. 2006. Maternal exposure to LPS induces hypomyelination in the internal capsule and programmed cell death in the deep gray matter in newborn rats. *Pediatr Res* 59 (3):428–33.

Rubin, D. B. 1974. Estimating causal effects of treatments in randomized and nonrandomized studies. *J Educ Psychol* 66 (5):688–701.

Rubin, D. B. 1997. Estimating causal effects from large data sets using propensity scores. *Ann Intern Med* 127 (8 Pt 2):757–63.

Rubin, D. B. 2007. The design versus the analysis of observational studies for causal effects: Parallels with the design of randomized trials. *Stat Med* 26 (1):20–36.

Russell, B. A. W. 1913. On the notion of cause. *Proceedings of the Aristotelian Society,* New Series. Vol. 13, pp. 1–26.

Russo, F. 2009. Variational causal claims in epidemiology. *Perspect Biol Med* 52 (4):540–54.

Russo, F. and J. Williamson, eds. 2007a. *Causality and Probability in the Sciences.* Texts in Philosophy, Vol. 5. London, UK: College Publications.

Russo, F. and J. Williamson. 2007b. Interpreting causality in the health sciences. *Int Stud Philos Sci* 21 (2):157–70.

Russo, F. and J. Williamson. 2011a. Epistemic causality and evidence-based medicine. *Hist Phil Life Sci* 3:563–82.

Russo, F. and J. Williamson. 2011b. Generic versus single-case causality: The case of autopsy. *Eur J Phil Sci* 1:47–69.

Russo, F. and J. Williamson. 2012. EnviroGenomarkers: The interplay between mechanisms and difference making in establishing causal claims. *Med Stud: Int J History, Philos Ethics Med Allied Sci* 3 (4):249–62.

Sackett, D. L. and W. M. Rosenberg. 1995. The need for evidence-based medicine. *J R Soc Med* 88 (11):620–4.

Salmon, W. C. 1993. Causality: Production and propagation. In *Causation*, edited by E. Sosa and M. Tooley, 154–71. Oxford, UK: Oxford University Press.

Salmon, W. C. 1997. Causality and explanation: A reply to two critiques. *Philos Sci* 64 (3):461–77.

Salmon, W. C. 1984. *Scientific Explanation and the Causal Structure of the World.* Princeton, NJ: Princeton University Press.

Salmon, W. C. 1998. *Causality and Explanation.* New York, NY: Oxford University Press.

Samuels, S. W. 1998. Philosophic perspectives: Community, communications, and occupational disease causation. *Int J Health Serv* 28 (1):153–64.

Sandin, S., P. Lichtenstein, R. Kuja-Halkola, H. Larsson, C. M. Hultman, and A. Reichenberg. 2014. The familial risk of autism. *JAMA* 311 (17):1770–7.

Sartwell, P. E. 1960. "On the methodology of investigations of etiologic factors in chronic diseases" – Further comments. *J Chronic Dis* 11:61–3.

Savitz, D. A. 2003. *Interpreting Epidemiologic Evidence.* Oxford, UK: Oxford University Press.

Schendel, D. and T. K. Bhasin. 2008. Birth weight and gestational age characteristics of children with autism, including a comparison with other developmental disabilities. *Pediatrics* 121 (6):1155–64.

Scheutz, F. and S. Poulsen. 1999. Determining causation in epidemiology. *Community Dent Oral Epidemiol* 27 (3):161–70.

Schubeler, D. 2015. Function and information content of DNA methylation. *Nature* 517 (7534):321–6.

Schulte, P. A. and F. P. Perera. 1993. *Molecular Epidemiology. Principles and Practices.* San Diego, CA: Academic Press.

Searle, J. R. 1984. *Minds, Brains, and Science: The 1984 Reith Lectures.* Cambridge, MA: Harvard University Press.

Semmelweis, I. 1983. *The Etiology, Concept, and Prophylaxis of Childbed Fever.* Translated by K. Codell Carter. Madison, WI: University of Wisconsin Press.

Severinsen, M. 2001. Principles behind definitions of diseases – A criticism of the principle of disease mechanism and the development of a pragmatic alternative. *Theor Med Bioeth* 22 (4):319–36.

Sjoberg, L., L. E. Holm, H. Ullen, and Y. Brandberg. 2004. Tanning and risk perception in adolescents. *Health Risk & Society* 6 (1):81–94.

Skrabanek, P. 1994. The emptiness of the black box. *Epidemiology* 5 (5):553–5.

Sloman, S. A. and D. Lagnado. 2015. Causality in thought. *Annu Rev Psychol* 66:223–47.

Smith, G. D. 2001. Reflections on the limitations to epidemiology. *J Clin Epidemiol* 54 (4):325–31.

Spirtes, P., C. N. Glymour, and R. Scheines. 1993. *Causation, Prediction, and Search, Lecture Notes in Statistics.* New York, NY: Springer-Verlag.

Stampfer, M. J., G. A. Colditz, W. C. Willett, J. E. Manson, B. Rosner, F. E. Speizer, and C. H. Hennekens. 1991. Postmenopausal estrogen therapy and cardiovascular disease. Ten-year follow-up from the nurses' health study. *N Engl J Med* 325 (11):756–62.

Stampfer, M. J., W. C. Willett, G. A. Colditz, B. Rosner, F. E. Speizer, and C. H. Hennekens. 1985. A prospective study of postmenopausal estrogen therapy and coronary heart disease. *N Engl J Med* 313 (17):1044–9.

Stanley, F., E. Blair, and E. Alberman. 2000. *Cerebral Palsies: Epidemiology & Causal Pathways.* Vol. 151, Clinics in Developmental Medicine. London, UK: Mac Keith.

Stegenga, J. 2009. Robustness, discordance, and relevance. *Philos Sci* 76:650–61.

Stehbens, W. E. 1992. Causality in medical science with particular reference to heart disease and atherosclerosis. *Perspect Biol Med* 36 (1):97–119.

Susser, E. 2004. Eco-epidemiology: Thinking outside the black box. *Epidemiology* 15 (5):519–20; author reply 527–8.

Susser, M. 1977. Judgement and causal inference: Criteria in epidemiologic studies. *Am J Epidemiol* 105 (1):1–15.

Susser, M. 1986. The logic of Sir Karl Popper and the practice of epidemiology. *Am J Epidemiol* 124 (5):711–8.

Susser, M. 1991. What is a cause and how do we know one? A grammar for pragmatic epidemiology. *Am J Epidemiol* 133:635–48.

Susser, M. and E. Susser. 1996. Choosing a future for epidemiology: II. From black box to Chinese boxes and eco-epidemiology. *Am J Public Health* 86 (5):674–7.

Susser, M. W. 1973. Causal thinking in the health sciences – Concepts and strategies of epidemiology. New York, NY: Oxford University Press.

Sutton, A. J. and K. R. Abrams. 2001. Bayesian methods in meta-analysis and evidence synthesis. *Stat Methods Med Res* 10 (4):277–303.

Taubes, G. 1995. Epidemiology faces its limits. *Science* 269 (5221):164–9.

Thagard, P. 1999. *How Scientists Explain Disease.* Princeton, NJ: Princeton University Press.

Thagard, P. 2000. *Coherence in Thought and Action, Life and Mind.* Cambridge, MA: MIT Press.

Thagard, P. 2004. Causal inference in legal decision making: Explanatory coherence vs. Bayesian networks. *Appl Artif Intell* 18 (3–4):231–49.

Thagard, P. 2006. Evaluating explanations in law, science, and everyday life. *Curr Dir Psychol Sci* 15 (3):141–5.

Thagard, P. 2007. Coherence, truth, and the development of scientific knowledge. *Phil Sci* 74:28–47.

Thompson, W. D. 1991. Effect modification and the limits of biological inference from epidemiologic data. *J Clin Epidemiol* 44 (3):221–32.

Thygesen, L. C., G. S. Andersen, and H. Andersen. 2005. A philosophical analysis of the Hill criteria. *J Epidemiol Community Health* 59 (6):512–6.

Toombs, S. K. 1992. *The Meaning of Illness: A Phenomenological Account of the Different Perspectives of Physician and Patient, Philosophy and Medicine.* Dordrecht, Netherlands: Kluwer Academic Publishers.

Trichopoulos, D. 1995. The discipline of epidemiology. *Science* 269 (5229):1326.

Tulchinsky, T. H. and E. Varavikova. 2009. *The New Public Health.* 2nd ed. Waltham, MA: Elsevier/Academic Press.

Udensi, U. K. and P. B. Tchounwou. 2014. Dual effect of oxidative stress on leukemia cancer induction and treatment. *J Exp Clin Cancer Res* 33:106.

U.S. Surgeon General's Advisory Committee on Smoking and Health. 1964. *Smoking and Health; Report of the Advisory Committee to the Surgeon General of the Public Health Service, Public Health Service Publication no 1103.* Washington, DC: U.S. Department of Health, Education, and Welfare, Public Health Service; for sale by the Superintendent of Documents, U.S. Government Printing Office.

Urbach, P. 1993. The value of randomization and control in clinical trials. *Stat Med* 12 (15–16):1421–31.

van de Looij, Y., G. A. Lodygensky, J. Dean, F. Lazeyras, H. Hagberg, I. Kjellmer, C. Mallard, P. S. Huppi, and S. V. Sizonenko. 2012. High-field diffusion tensor imaging characterization of cerebral white matter injury in lipopolysaccharide-exposed fetal sheep. *Pediatr Res* 72 (3):285–92.

Vandenbroucke, J. P. 1998. Clinical investigation in the 20th century: The ascendancy of numerical reasoning. *Lancet* 352 (Suppl 2):SII12–6.

Vandenbroucke, J. P., A. Broadbent, and N. Pearce. 2016. Causality and causal inference in epidemiology: The need for a pluralistic approach. *Int J Epidemiol* 45 (6):1776–86.

VanderWeele, T. J. 2015. *Explanation in Causal Inference: Methods for Mediation and Interaction.* New York, NY: Oxford University Press.

Van Fraassen Bas, C. 1980. *The Scientific Image.* Oxford, UK: Oxford University Press.

Vannucci, S. J. and H. Hagberg. 2004. Hypoxia-ischemia in the immature brain. *J Exp Biol* 207 (Pt 18):3149–54.

Vargas, D. L., C. Nascimbene, C. Krishnan, A. W. Zimmerman, and C. A. Pardo. 2005. Neuroglial activation and neuroinflammation in the brain of patients with autism. *Ann Neurol* 57 (1):67–81.

Verney, C., I. Pogledic, V. Biran, H. Adle-Biassette, C. Fallet-Bianco, and P. Gressens. 2012. Microglial reaction in axonal crossroads is a hallmark of noncystic periventricular white matter injury in very preterm infants. *J Neuropathol Exp Neurol* 71 (3):251–64.

Vincent, C. 2003. Understanding and responding to adverse events. *N Engl J Med* 348 (11):1051–6.

Vincent, C. A. 2004. Analysis of clinical incidents: A window on the system not a search for root causes. *Qual Saf Health Care* 13 (4):242–3.

Vineis, P. and F. Perera. 2007. Molecular epidemiology and biomarkers in etiologic cancer research: The new in light of the old. *Cancer Epidemiol Biomarkers Prev* 16 (10):1954–65.

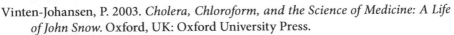

Vinten-Johansen, P. 2003. *Cholera, Chloroform, and the Science of Medicine: A Life of John Snow*. Oxford, UK: Oxford University Press.

Volpe, J. J. 2009. Brain injury in premature infants: A complex amalgam of destructive and developmental disturbances. *Lancet Neurol* 8 (1):110–24.

Waddington, C. H. 1957. *The Strategy of the Genes; a Discussion of Some Aspects of Theoretical Biology*. London, UK: Allen & Unwin.

Waldron, L. 2018. Statistical issues in population health informatics. In *Population Health Nformatics*, edited by A. Joshi, L. Thorpe and L. Waldron, 145–60. Burlington, MA: Jones & Bartlett.

Ward, A. 2009a. Causal criteria and the problem of complex causation. *Med Health Care Philos* 12 (3):333–43.

Ward, A. C. 2009b. The role of causal criteria in causal inferences: Bradford Hill's "aspects of association." *Epidemiol Perspect Innov* 6:2.

Webb, P. and C. Bain. 2011. *Essential Epidemiology: An Introduction for Students and Health Professionals*. 2nd ed. Cambridge Medicine. Cambridge, England: Cambridge University Press.

Weber, E. 2009. How probabilistic causation can account for the use of mechanistic evidence. *Int Stud Philos Sci* 23 (3):277–95.

Weed, D. L. 1985. An epidemiological application of Popper's method. *J Epidemiol Community Health* 39 (4):277–85.

Weed, D. L. 1986. On the logic of causal inference. *Am J Epidemiol* 123 (6):965–79.

Weed, D. L. 1997. On the use of causal criteria. *Int J Epidemiol* 26 (6):1137–41.

Weed, D. L. 2008. Truth, epidemiology, and general causation. *Brooklyn Law Rev* 73 (3):943–57.

Weed, D. W. 1988. Causal criteria and Popperian refutation. In *Causal Inference*, edited by K. J. Rothman, 15–32. Chestnut Hill, MA: Epidemiology Resources, Inc.

Wenig, K. 1998/99. War rudolf virchow ein gegner der evolutionstheorie? *Philosophia Scientiae* (S2):211–29.

Wetzel, L. 2018. Types and tokens. In *The Stanford Encyclopedia of Philosophy (Fall 2018 ed.)*, edited by E. N. Zalta.

Whitehead, A. N. 1929 (1960). *Process and Reality, an Essay in Cosmology, Gifford Lectures*. New York, NY: Free Press.

Williamson, J. 2005. *Bayesian Nets and Causality: Philosophical and Computational Foundations*. New York, NY: Oxford University Press.

Williamson, J. 2006. Dispositional versus epistemic causality. *Minds Mach: J Artif Intell, Philos Cogn Sci* 16 (3):259–76.

Williamson, J. 2009. Probabilistic theories. In *The Oxford Handbook of Causation*, edited by H. Beebee, C. Hitchcock and P. Menzies, 185–212. Oxford, UK: Oxford University Press.

Williamson, J. 2011a. Mechanistic theories of causality part I. *Philos Compass* 6 (6):421–32.

Williamson, J. 2011b. Mechanistic theories of causality part II. *Philos Compass* 6 (6):433–44.

Williamson, T. 2000. *Knowledge and Its Limits*. Oxford, UK: Oxford University Press.

Wilson, E. O. 1980. *Sociobiology*. The abridged edition. Cambridge, MA: Belknap Press.

Wilson, M. A., J. W. Baurley, D. C. Thomas, and D. V. Conti. 2010. Complex system approaches to genetic analysis Bayesian approaches. *Adv Genet* 72:47–71.

Wilson, P. W., R. J. Garrison, and W. P. Castelli. 1985. Postmenopausal estrogen use, cigarette smoking, and cardiovascular morbidity in women over 50. The Framingham Study. *N Engl J Med* 313 (17):1038–43.

Woodward, J. 2003. Making things happen – A theory of causal explanation.

Woodward, J. 2009. Agency and interventionist theories. In *The Oxford Handbook of Causation*, edited by H. Beebee, C. Hitchcock and P. Menzies, 234–62. Oxford, UK: Oxford University Press.

Woodward, J. 2014. A functional account of causation; or, a defense of the legitimacy of causal thinking by reference to the only standard that matters – Usefulness (as opposed to metaphysics or agreement with intuitive judgment). *Philos Sci* 81 (5):691–713.

Woodward, J. 2017. Scientific explanation. In *The Stanford Encyclopedia of Philosophy*, edited by E. N. Zalta.

Worrall, J. 2007. Why there's no cause to randomize. *Br J Philos Sci* 58 (3):451–88.

Worrall, J. 2011. Causality in medicine: Getting back to the Hill top. *Prev Med* 53 (4–5):235–8.

Wright, L. 1976. *Teleological Explanations*. Berkeley, CA: University of California Press.

Yanni, D., S. J. Korzeniewski, E. N. Allred, R. N. Fichorova, T. M. O'Shea, K. Kuban, O. Dammann, and A. Leviton. 2017. Both antenatal and postnatal inflammation contribute information about the risk of brain damage in extremely preterm newborns. *Pediatr Res* 82 (4):691–6.

Yarmolinsky, J., K. H. Wade, R. C. Richmond, R. J. Langdon, C. J. Bull, K. M. Tilling, C. L. Relton, S. J. Lewis, G. Davey Smith, and R. M. Martin. 2018. Causal inference in cancer epidemiology: What is the role of Mendelian randomization? *Cancer Epidemiol Biomarkers Prev* 27 (9):995–1010.

Yerushalmy, J. and C. E. Palmer. 1959. On the methodology of investigations of etiologic factors in chronic diseases. *J Chronic Dis* 10 (1):27–40.

Young, J. O. 2018. The coherence theory of truth. In *The Stanford Encyclopedia of Philosophy*, edited by E. N. Zalta. Stanford, CA: Metaphysics Research Lab, Stanford University.

Zikopoulos, B. and H. Barbas. 2013. Altered neural connectivity in excitatory and inhibitory cortical circuits in autism. *Front Hum Neurosci* 7:609.

Zimmerman, A. W., H. Jyonouchi, A. M. Comi, S. L. Connors, S. Milstien, A. Varsou, and M. P. Heyes. 2005. Cerebrospinal fluid and serum markers of inflammation in autism. *Pediatr Neurol* 33 (3):195–201.

INDEX

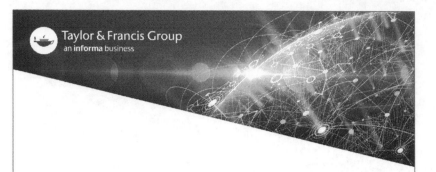